MENOPAUSE

**Questions
you
have
... Answers
you
need**

Other Books in This Series
From the People's Medical Society

MENOPAUSE

Questions
you
have
...Answers
you
need

By Annette Thevenin Doran

≡People's Medical Society®

Allentown, Pennsylvania

The People's Medical Society is a nonprofit consumer health organization dedicated to the principles of better, more responsive and less expensive medical care. Organized in 1983, the People's Medical Society puts previously unavailable medical information into the hands of consumers so that they can make informed decisions about their own health care.

Membership in the People's Medical Society is $20 a year and includes a subscription to the *People's Medical Society Newsletter.* For information, write to the People's Medical Society, 462 Walnut Street, Allentown, PA 18102, or call 610-770-1670.

This and other People's Medical Society publications are available for quantity purchase at discount. Contact the People's Medical Society for details.

Many of the designations used by manufacturers and sellers to distinguish their products are claimed as trademarks. Where those designations appear in this book and the People's Medical Society was aware of a trademark claim, the designations have been printed in initial capital letters (e.g., Premarin).

© 1999 by the People's Medical Society
Printed in the United States of America

Library of Congress Cataloging-in-Publication Data
Thevenin Doran, Annette, 1960–
       Menopause : questions you have . . . answers you need /
    by Annette Thevenin Doran.
          p. cm.
       Includes bibliographical references and index.
       ISBN 1-882606-45-0
       1. Menopause—Miscellanea.   I. Title.
    RG186.T48   1999
    618.1'75—dc21   98-31192
                                                            CIP

1 2 3 4 5 6 7 8 9 0
First printing, January 1999

CONTENTS

INTRODUCTION

You may not believe it, but menopause is not a disease. Of course, you would never know this if all the information you got was from magazines, radio talk shows and newspaper advertisements for products and programs intended to "cure" this "dreaded curse." There are even doctors, usually gynecologists, who "specialize" in menopause—often touting their approaches the same way an oncologist might promote a cancer treatment.

But menopause is not a disease. It's as normal and natural as puberty. It's something that every woman experiences (unless her life is cut short), some earlier or later than others, some with more difficulty than others.

For centuries, women dealt with menopause in a variety of ways. Some used folk or home remedies to deal with the often annoying symptoms—such as hot flashes, sleeplessness and mood swings—that menopause sometimes brings. Others visited shamans, witch doctors or spiritualists to help conquer their discomfort. Today, with the better understanding science now has of the process of menopause, women often visit physicians who have a whole arsenal of medicinal and non-medicinal approaches to treat menopausal symptoms. And of course, the leading treatment is hormone replacement therapy (HRT), which has spawned much controversy and debate.

Surprisingly, most women know very little about menopause. Sure, they know it is inevitable. Yes, they realize that the menstrual cycle ends. And there's hardly a woman who hasn't heard of or experienced a hot flash. But very few women know what is actually happening to their bodies, why certain discomforts or symptoms occur and, more important, what their options are for coping with and dealing with menopause.

That is exactly why we have written and published this book. *Menopause: Questions You Have ... Answers You Need* is designed not only to help you better understand what is happening to your body during menopause but also to aid you in making the important decisions you may face in dealing with its symptoms and menopause-related health conditions.

From HRT to foods that relieve symptoms and help prevent specific health conditions, it's all covered in the pages that follow. Using our popular question-and-answer format, we have attempted to present the information you need in a logical, easy-to-understand way. And what you will be reading is not hype or opinion. The information contained in these pages comes directly from the most authoritative medical studies.

Even more important is the fact that we have no medical bias. Our goal is to present you with the facts and information and let you make the decisions. That has always been the hallmark of the People's Medical Society.

So use this book as a tool and a guide to menopause. And know that the better you understand what's happening to your body and what your treatment options are, the more likely you'll be to take charge of your own health.

CHARLES B. INLANDER
President
People's Medical Society

MENOPAUSE

Questions
you
have
. . . Answers
you
need

Terms printed in boldface can be found in the glossary, beginning on page 165. Only the first mention of the word in the text will be boldfaced.

We have tried to use male and female pronouns in an egalitarian manner throughout the book. Any imbalance in usage has been in the interest of readability.

1 MENOPAUSE BASICS

Q: What is **menopause?**

A: Technically speaking, menopause is a medical term that means the normal and complete cessation of the **menstrual cycle**, including both **ovulation** (the release of an unfertilized egg from the **ovaries**—two almond-shaped glands alongside the **uterus** that contain unfertilized egg cells) and menstrual periods. In this usage, menopause is a discrete, one-time event: a woman's last menstrual period.

In everyday usage, however, the word *menopause* can refer to the months before and the years after the last period. Women often use the phrase "change of life" to describe menopause, and doctors may call it the **climacteric**.

Menopause is an inevitable phase of life. Every woman eventually experiences it unless her life is cut short.

Q: At what age does menopause take place?

A: Menopause usually takes place between the ages of 45 and 55, although some women experience their last periods in their 60s, and others in their 30s.

New research shows that genetic factors may determine the age at which a woman reaches menopause. In a British study of women ages 45 to 54, those women whose mothers had experienced early menopause were six times more likely to reach menopause early (between ages 40 and 45) or even prematurely (before age 40) than women whose mothers reached menopause after age 45.

Q: What are the signals that menopause is approaching?

A: Disrupted menstrual cycles and irregular periods are common flags of its onset. But before we can examine the "classic" signs and symptoms of menopause, we need to take a look at the female reproductive system and the role of **hormones** in this system.

THE FEMALE REPRODUCTIVE SYSTEM

Q: OK, let's start. What are the structures, and how do they work?

A: A woman's external sex organs are contained in an area called the **vulva**. The external sex organs located in the vulva area are the **labia majora** (outer lips), the **labia minora** (inner lips), the introitus (vaginal opening), the **clitoris** and the **Bartholin's glands** (two small glands located slightly inside the vaginal opening).

Q: Stop right there. What do these parts of the anatomy do?

A: The two folds of fleshy tissue on the outermost part of the vulva, the labia majora and labia minora, help protect the vulva. The labia minora also contain sweat and oil glands, which help to discharge waste. The introitus allows menstrual flow or a baby to pass out of the body, and it's the area that the penis enters during intercourse. Located between the labia and the top of the vulva, the clitoris is highly sensitive to the touch; indeed, its only known function is for sexual pleasure. The Bartholin's glands secrete fluids that provide lubrication during sexual excitement.

The **urethra**—which is not actually part of the reproductive system—conveys urine from the bladder to the outside.

Q: What are the internal structures?

A: A woman's internal reproductive organs include the **vagina**, the uterus, the **fallopian tubes** and the ovaries. The vagina is a stretchable passage between a woman's vulva and her **cervix** (the narrow lower portion, or neck, of the uterus) and uterus.

The uterus is a pear-shaped organ about the size of a tennis ball. The inner lining of the uterus is called the **endometrium**, which nourishes a fertilized egg and plays a role in hormone production. The fallopian tubes extend from the top of each side of the uterus. Each fallopian tube ends near an ovary. The outer edge of each tube is funnel-shaped, with tassel-like projections that draw an egg from the ovary into the tube. The contractions of the fallopian tube and the movements of the cilia—fine hairlike fringes—move the egg toward the uterus.

Q: Back to the ovaries—what role do they play in this system?

A: Attached by ligaments to each side of the uterus and to the walls of the pelvis, the ovaries produce the hormones **estrogen** and **progesterone**, as well as a small amount of **testosterone**. Each ovary has thousands of **follicles**, tiny sacs that hold immature eggs. As an egg—or **ovum**, the female reproductive cell—matures, the follicle grows.

HORMONES AND YOUR BODY

Q: OK—on to hormones. What is a hormone?

A: A hormone is a complex chemical secreted by certain glands in the body. Hormones act as chemical messengers, traveling through the bloodstream and controlling the action of a specific organ (called the target organ) or group of cells. The growth hormone, for example, controls the growth of bones in the body. In the female body, the hormone estrogen is just one of several hormones that control the reproductive process.

Hormones are often assisted by hormonelike fatty acids called **mediators**, which are produced in tiny amounts in body tissues such as the uterus. If hormones are the chemical messengers, the mediators are the chemicals that actually do the job. **Prostaglandin**, for example, is a mediator. It causes contractions in the uterus during **menstruation** and during the labor phase of pregnancy.

Q: What produces the hormones?

A: The actions of many interrelated organs and glands. Technically known as the **endocrine system**, this network manufactures hormones and releases them into the bloodstream.

Q: What role does the endocrine system play in reproduction?

A: The reproductive part of the endocrine system is controlled by the **hypothalamus**, a small but powerful gland in the brain. The hypothalamus works in conjunction with the **pituitary gland** (a pebble-size gland beneath the hypothalamus), the **adrenal glands** (two secretory organs perched atop the kidneys), the uterus and the ovaries to regulate the menstrual cycle throughout a woman's child-bearing years. These components are also responsible for starting **puberty**.

Each month, the hypothalamus produces and sends **gonadotropin-releasing hormones** (also called releasing factors) to the pituitary gland. The pituitary gland, in turn, manufactures two hormones called **gonadotropins** (hormones that stimulate the ovaries).

Q: How do hormones specifically affect the body?

A: Hormones are responsible for every cycle of the body: growth during childhood; the physical transformation from girl to woman; the preparation of the body for childbearing, pregnancy and labor; the gradual cessation of menstruation; and the postmenopausal years. A normal infant girl is born with all the elements of the female reproductive system, which gradually develops through late childhood and begins functioning as she reaches **menarche** (her first menstrual period) sometime between the ages of 10 and 16. Similarly, the reproductive system slowly stops functioning in midlife as a woman approaches menopause.

Q: Speaking of menstruation, can we talk about the specific hormones and the roles they play in that process?

A: Certainly. As you probably know, the menstrual cycle is a pattern of fertility and infertility that usually repeats itself monthly. The menstrual cycle can last from 21 to 35 days, depending upon the individual woman. Indeed, the length may also change from month to month.

The four hormones that regulate the menstrual cycle are progesterone, estrogen, **luteinizing hormone (LH)** and **follicle-stimulating hormone (FSH)**.

The menstrual cycle can be divided into two parts: before ovulation and after ovulation. During the first half of the menstrual cycle, three major steps occur.

- Menstruation takes place, usually from day 1 to day 5.

- An egg matures in a follicle of an ovary. The maturing is caused by the release of FSH from the pituitary gland between day 5 and day 7.

- The lining of the uterus begins to thicken, caused by the release of estrogen from the follicle between day 7 and day 11.

At ovulation, the ripe egg is released from the follicle. Ovulation is triggered by the release of LH from the pituitary gland about 14 days before the start of the next menstrual cycle.

 Q: What happens then?

A: During the second half of the menstrual cycle, three major steps occur.

- The ripe egg is swept into the fallopian tube, from which it travels toward the uterus.

- The lining of the uterus continues to thicken. After ovulation, the follicle develops into the **corpus luteum**, a small, yellow lump that secretes progesterone. Together with estrogen secreted by the ovaries, progesterone thickens the lining of the uterus, which becomes engorged with blood to prepare for the implantation of a fertilized egg.

- If fertilization doesn't take place, the pituitary gland shuts down the production of FSH and LH in response to the high levels of estrogen and progesterone in the bloodstream. This causes the corpus luteum to break down, and estrogen and progesterone production decreases. The lower hormone levels cause the lining of the uterus to break down and flow out through the vagina as menstrual bleeding, and the cycle begins again.

Q: **Back to menopause—isn't estrogen the key to this process?**

A: Yes. The menstrual cycle halts when the female body no longer produces enough estrogen—primarily a female or feminizing hormone, although men do produce it in much smaller amounts.

And scientifically speaking, the word *estrogen* is a generic term. There are actually three types of estrogen: **estradiol**, **estrone** and **estriol**.

The most potent form of estrogen, estradiol is manufactured by the ovaries and is part of the intricate biological system that results in the normal monthly ovulatory cycle. Estrone, a low-level estrogen, is made in the body's fatty tissues. Although produced at much lower levels than estradiol, estrone plays a role in building strong bones both before and after menopause. The third estrogen, estriol, is relatively weak and is generated when estradiol and estrone are used in the body.

Q: **What exactly is the role of estrogen in the female body again?**

A: As a group, the three estrogens have fundamental tasks. First, estrogens function in the development of the breasts, ovaries and uterus from the time of adolescence through the reproductive years. Second, estrogens function in the menstrual cycle itself, as we've already seen.

Q: Does estrogen affect only the reproductive cycle?

A: No. Estrogen affects other areas of the body, too. The tissues in the cervix, vagina and bladder are sensitive to estrogen levels in the bloodstream. Estrogen helps bones absorb calcium, keeping **bone mass** high and bones strong. And in the blood itself, estrogen raises the levels of **HDL (high-density lipoprotein)**, the so-called good cholesterol, while lowering the levels of **LDL (low-density lipoprotein)**, the so-called bad cholesterol.

Q: Does estrogen do its work alone?

A: No. Estrogen is assisted by progesterone, another female hormone produced by the ovaries. Briefly, in the process of reproduction, estrogen's primary task is to build up the lining of the uterus to receive a fertilized egg. If an egg is fertilized, progesterone prepares the uterus to accept the egg so that the egg can grow. If the egg is unfertilized, progesterone assists in shedding the uterine lining, which, as you know, causes the normal bleeding called menstruation.

From the time a woman's menstrual cycle becomes regular until her childbearing years end (generally between ages 45 and 55), her body is on a monthly cycle of hormone release and response, as we've described.

CHANGES IN THE MENOPAUSAL YEARS

Q: It has been six months since my last period. Am I menopausal?

A: The answer isn't so simple. You could be perimenopausal (the time just before menopause), or you could be menopausal. "Classic" menopausal symptoms—including **hot flashes**, **night sweats** or excessive sweating, **palpitations**, vaginal dryness, irregular or prolonged periods, and mood swings—can suggest that you are beyond the perimenopausal stage. However, some perimenopausal women can have menopausal discomfort.

Q: What happens during **perimenopause?**

A: The term *perimenopause* refers to the years immediately before menopause. Between two and six years before your last menstrual period, your ovaries have difficulty producing viable egg follicles. The common misconception is that women run out of eggs. This isn't the case. Instead, ovarian function declines. The ovaries simply fail to respond to the command by FSH to "ripen an egg." The ovaries release eggs irregularly instead of monthly. Eventually, no more egg follicles ripen, and the woman stops ovulating.

Most women enter perimenopause by their late 40s. Because natural menopause can occur by age 45, some women enter perimenopause by their late 30s.

Q: Do the ovaries stop producing estrogen during perimenopause?

A: No. During this time, the ovaries continue to produce estrogen—partly out of habit and partly in a final attempt to keep the reproductive process going. Also during this time, production of the second important female hormone, progesterone, becomes erratic. So while the estrogen in your body continues to build up the endometrium to accept a fertilized egg, menstruation occurs only if progesterone is present. When ovulation becomes irregular, your body does not have progesterone to cause regular menstrual periods.

Q: So menstrual periods become unpredictable, right?

A: Yes. They usually become less frequent, although some women have more frequent periods just before menopause. Menstruation can disappear for several months and then reappear; the duration and flow can also change. For most women, changes in their menstrual cycles are the first flag that menopause is approaching.

Q: Is pregnancy still possible in the perimenopausal years?

A: Yes. Technically, you are still in your reproductive years. Although menstrual periods may be irregular, your body is still releasing eggs, and pregnancy is possible.

Q: How long do irregular periods last?

A: Irregular menstrual cycles can occur from a few months to several years before menstruation finally stops. A few women, though, experience no menstrual irregularities at all. And up to 20 percent of perimenopausal women experience the discomforts associated with menopause itself, particularly hot flashes and vaginal dryness.

Q: How can I know for sure if I'm perimenopausal or menopausal?

A: If you are in your 30s or 40s and are having menstrual irregularities, your medical practitioner may suspect that you are entering your perimenopausal years. And *suspect* is the key word here. As we've said, the presence of meno-pausal symptoms can suggest that you are beyond the perimenopausal stage, but some perimenopausal women can have menopausal symptoms.

A doctor can confirm that you have entered menopause if (a) you are over age 40 and have gone 12 consecutive months without a menstrual period or (b) your **follicle-stimulating hormone test** shows FSH levels above 40 I.U./ml. (international units per milliliter of blood).

Q: So there's a test that measures FSH levels. Are there other tests as well?

A: Yes. A blood test can measure FSH levels, and other medical tests and procedures can confirm whether a woman is perimenopausal or menopausal. Let's look at these now.

- *FSH test.* **FSH test** is a blood test that measures the amount of follicle-stimulating hormone, which, you'll remember, is the hormone that tells dormant, or immature, egg cells in the ovaries to ripen. As you near menopause, your ovaries respond more slowly to FSH, so the pituitary gland in the brain works overtime to make more of this hormone. Levels of FSH in the bloodstream rise.

  In a premenopausal woman, FSH levels are lower than 30 I.U./ml. Levels higher than 30 I.U./ml. indicate that you are perimenopausal and that menopause is imminent. Eventually, your levels pass the 40 I.U./ml. mark—sometimes nearing 1,000. Once they reach 40 I.U./ml., FSH levels rarely fall below that measurement. Thus, exceeding the 40 I.U./ml. mark is one sign of the onset of menopause. Another, of course, is cessation of menstrual periods.

- *Progesterone challenge test.* Used alone or to confirm the results of an FSH test, the **progesterone challenge test** determines if irregular periods are caused by insufficient progesterone. In this test, you take **progestin** (a synthetic or natural form of progesterone) for one week a month for several months. If progestin makes menstrual periods regular and normal in flow, then you have probably entered perimenopause.

- *Endometrial biopsy.* In an **endometrial biopsy** (usually an in-office procedure), the physician takes a small sample of your endometrium. The sample is examined microscopically, measured for thickness and analyzed for the presence of abnormal cells. This biopsy is one way to check irregular bleeding and make sure that it is not due to **hyperplasia** (a proliferation of cells in the endometrium that can set the stage for cancer) or another health condition.

Q: If my FSH levels are high, can I give up birth control without getting pregnant?

A: Most doctors recommend that you wait 12 months after your last period before giving up birth control.

COMMON MENOPAUSAL SYMPTOMS

Q: What are some of the signs that I may be entering menopause?

A: As we've said before, shorter or irregular periods are the first signals of hormonal changes that lead to the transition.

Q: So these hormonal changes are key?

A: Yes, in a manner of speaking. As time goes by, FSH and LH no longer have any effect on the ovaries.

Sheldon H. Cherry, M.D., and Carolyn D. Runowicz, M.D., authors of *The Menopause Book,* call this situation *ovarian shutdown,* and they say it's the cause of menopause. Once out of business, the ovaries stop producing estradiol.

Q: What happens when the ovaries shut down?

A: In response to the fall in estrogen levels, **atrophic** (degenerative) changes begin to affect the body. Estrogen-sensitive organs become smaller, and estrogen-sensitive tissues waste away. The uterus and ovaries shrink. The breasts lose layers of fat and glandular tissue. The endometrium, no longer needed to receive a fertilized egg, thins. The vaginal walls, no longer in demand as a birth canal, become thinner and less elastic. The tissue of the urethra becomes thin. Bone mass begins to decrease. The skin becomes thinner and loses some elasticity. It also loses **collagen**, which acts as a padding under the skin and makes the skin more resilient. In summary, the physical growth and development that estrogen spurred and sustained in adolescence are reversed.

Q: What effects do these changes have?

A: Each woman is affected differently. Some women, for example, experience dry and easily irritated vaginal walls several months after menopause, while others never notice any changes in vaginal health.

As you can imagine, the amount of estrogen the body continues to produce is the reason for the woman-to-woman variation. While the ovaries, a woman's major source of estradiol, drastically curtail estrogen production at menopause, some other tissues may compensate. For example, fat cells convert a hormone called androstenedione, produced by the adrenal glands, into estrone. Women with ample body fat produce more estrone than thin women. The continued presence of estrogen after menopause (although not at the same levels as in the premenopausal years) may be one reason why some women experience fewer atrophic changes than others, particularly the loss of bone mass related to **osteoporosis**. (We talk more about osteoporosis in chapters 2 and 3.)

Q: How long does it take for these changes to develop?

A: Atrophic changes take years to develop, if they develop at all. Conversely, menopausal discomforts, such as hot flashes, insomnia and night sweats, can occur immediately after estradiol levels in the blood decrease. These discomforts are signs of the hormonal upheaval the body is experiencing. As the body becomes accustomed to its new estrogen levels (usually within two to five years), menopausal discomforts often fade away.

Q: Does every woman experience discomfort from menopause?

A: About 25 percent of women glide through menopause, noticing the cessation of their menstrual periods but experiencing few side effects. The other 75 percent experience the effects of decreased estrogen levels in the form of hot flashes, sleepless nights and mood swings. These so-called classic signs of menopause may be fleeting, manageable or intolerable, depending upon the woman.

Q: I've heard about something called **vasomotor symptoms.** Can you explain what these are?

A: Certainly. First off, let us say that in medical parlance, there are two common types of menopausal symptoms: vasomotor symptoms and **genitourinary symptoms**.

Vasomotor symptoms are those related to the nerves and muscles that open and close blood vessels. Vasomotor problems usually disappear within five years after menopause.

Hot flashes are the most common vasomotor symptom, as well as the most common complaint of menopausal women. Otherwise known as a **hot flush**, a hot flash is a sensation of intense warmth and a pink flush in the head, neck and upper body. A hot flash can last from a few seconds to two minutes. Some women report that their flashes last up to one hour. Typically, the hot flash is accompanied by heavy perspiration and rapid pulse and followed by chills and shivering.

Q: What causes hot flashes?

A: Current thought is that they are related to two things. The first is the *abrupt* drop in ovarian estrogen (estradiol) that occurs once you enter menopause. Scientists believe that hot flashes are due to sudden drops in estradiol levels rather than low estradiol levels in general. This is why they suspect that women who have had **surgical menopause** (both ovaries surgically removed) tend to have the most severe hot flashes for years after menopause.

Q: So what is the second cause?

A: A disruption of the body's thermostat (the hypo-thalamus) by gonadotropins appears to be the second cause of hot flashes. The thermostat usually works like this: When your body's temperature is high—perhaps because you have a fever—the hypothalamus releases signals that instruct the body to dilate (widen) blood vessels, so more blood travels to the skin and transfers excess heat. A high temperature alerts the hypothalamus to activate sweat glands under the skin, cooling your body. When your body temperature is low—

perhaps you've been outdoors in the cold weather—the hypothalamus tells the blood vessels to constrict (narrow) to reduce heat loss. The gland instructs your body to produce heat through shivering.

During menopause, this thermostat may go awry. It acts as though your body temperature has increased (when it has not), thus causing the body to start the cool-down process by transferring excess heat to the skin and activating the sweat glands. Hot flashes and drenching sweats are the result. During a hot flash, skin temperature can increase anywhere from 8° to 12°F.

Q: I know you said that hot flashes generally disappear within five years of menopause. But do they ever last longer? Decades?

A: While most women's hot flashes disappear within five years of menopause, about 25 percent of women experience hot flashes for six to 10 years, and 10 percent have hot flashes 10 years after their last periods. Hot flashes may be mild or intense—a daily fleeting sensation of warmth or a series (up to 50 a day) of sweats and chills that may disrupt sleep and lead to exhaustion and irritability.

Q: Are you saying that hot flashes can lead to other problems?

A: Yes. Sleep problems are often caused by hot flashes. Women with frequent hot flashes may repeatedly awaken because they feel warm, even sweaty. Over the course of time, such disrupted sleep can cause memory lapses and feelings of anxiety. This can lead to mood swings and further anxiety, says Susan M. Love, M.D., in *Dr. Susan Love's Hormone Book.*

Q: Are there other vasomotor symptoms?

A: **Formication**, the sensation of something crawling on your skin, is a vasomotor effect, as are itchiness and dizziness.

Q: What are genitourinary symptoms?

A: Genitourinary symptoms usually develop later than vasomotor symptoms. Rather than occurring in response to plummeting estrogen levels, genitourinary symptoms develop after estrogen levels have remained low for months or years. These symptoms, including dryness, itchiness and a sensation of burning in the vagina, are reflections of the atrophic changes that occur in the body once the ovaries stop making estradiol.

You see, when estradiol levels decline, the cervix slows down its production of cervical mucus, making the vagina drier. As noted earlier, the vaginal walls also thin. When this happens, bumping or rubbing the walls of the vagina—say, during sexual intercourse—may cause light bleeding. Vaginal dryness can make intercourse unpleasant or downright painful.

Q: Are there other genitourinary symptoms?

A: More frequent urination is another symptom. It results when the tissue lining of the urethra shrinks and becomes brittle after estrogen levels fall. Some women experience **nocturia** (excessive urination at night). Occasionally, urination may be painful.

Also, vaginal infections (vaginitis) and urinary tract infections become more frequent. The vagina's pH (acid balance) changes after menopause and becomes less acidic, thus making the vagina more hospitable to bacteria that cause vaginal infections. The thinning and shortening of the urinary tract (two of the atrophic changes caused by low estrogen levels) make it easier for bacteria to reach the urethra and flourish there.

Q: That's a lot of symptoms! Are there any more?

A: Possibly. Symptoms not classified as either vasomotor or genitourinary include mood changes, depression, irritability, anxiety and the inability to concentrate. All have been blamed on biological changes that take place during the menopausal years. Just how much the lack of estrogen plays a role in these changes is a matter of lively debate.

Numerous studies have determined that in emotionally healthy women, menopause by itself does not cause depression. However, negative emotional feelings at menopause may be the result of having to cope with the symptoms we've been talking about, as well as fears of old age and other stresses that can contribute to depression.

PREMATURE MENOPAUSE

Q: I understand the changes in the menopausal years and the common menopausal symptoms. But I'd like to return to an earlier mention of surgical menopause. What is that?

A: First, let us say that about 9 percent of women experience menopause before the age of 40. This situation is known as **premature menopause**. Surgical removal of the ovaries (**oophorectomy**)—which results in what is called surgical menopause, or **artificial menopause**—is the most frequent cause of premature menopause. Without ovaries, your body no longer produces estradiol, and menopause immediately begins.

In the past, an oophorectomy was usually done along with a **hysterectomy** (surgical removal of the uterus). However, the practice is less common today, according to Love. Either the ovaries are left intact or only one ovary is removed.

Q: Why the switch in medical practice?

A: Your ovaries produce large amounts of estradiol during your reproductive years and smaller but important amounts of other estrogens for 10 to 20 years after menopause. Medical science is only just beginning to understand how valuable these other, nonestradiol estrogens can be in the postmenopausal years.

Q: Are menopausal symptoms severe with surgical menopause?

A: They can be. If your ovaries are still producing estradiol at the time they are surgically removed (and they probably are if you are under age 45), you will probably experience severe menopausal symptoms such as hot flashes. These symptoms often are more severe than those that accompany a natural, nonsurgical menopause because of the suddenness of the removal of the ovaries, writes Wulf H. Utian, M.D., in *Managing Your Menopause*. Generally, the more abrupt the drop in estrogen levels, the more intense the symptoms of menopause.

Q: If surgical removal of the ovaries is the most common cause of early menopause, what are the other causes?

A: Smoking can bring on early menopause, although doctors are not sure why. Utian points to two current theories: that some substance in cigarette smoke destroys

estrogen, and that the nicotine in cigarette smoke reduces the blood supply to the ovaries and causes them to prematurely fail.

Q: Are there other causes of early menopause?

A: Radiation therapy to treat pelvic cancer destroys the ovaries. Chemical therapy, or chemotherapy, to treat other cancers (such as breast cancer) can sometimes destroy egg follicles or ovaries.

Other theories about the cause of early menopause include the presence of an autoimmune disorder, in which the body produces antibodies that disturb the ovaries or destroy ovarian tissue. As mentioned earlier, genetics may also play a role. If your mother had an early menopause, you may have one, too. It may also be that some women are born with fewer egg follicles or that they have some condition that causes the body to stop producing estrogen while they are still young.

OVERVIEW OF HORMONE REPLACEMENT THERAPY

Q: So depending upon the woman, the menopausal years can be a time of menstrual irregularities and discomforts such as hot flashes and vaginal dryness. Does medical science have a treatment for any of this?

A: Hormone replacement therapy (HRT) is a medical treatment to alleviate short-term menopausal discomforts and to slow atrophic changes to estrogen-sensitive tissues. It is designed to supplement and/or replace the hormones that are produced in smaller and smaller amounts during and after menopause. More than 11 million women over age 45 use HRT annually. HRT is also known by several other names: **estrogen therapy (ET)**, **estrogen replacement therapy (ERT)** and **combined hormone therapy (CHT)** or **combination therapy**. (We should mention here that while these are forms of HRT, they are not necessarily synonymous terms. We talk more about this in chapter 3.)

Q: Is this the only way to treat menopausal symptoms?

A: No. HRT is just one way to treat symptoms. If you are among the 5 percent of women who have a stress-free menopause, you and your doctor may decide that you do not need medical treatment in the form of HRT or other prescription drugs. But if your menopausal symptoms are disruptive or intolerable, interfering with your sleep or lifestyle, you may decide that treatment is for you.

Some women decide to take HRT for a short time—one to five years—to ease them through the worst of their symptoms. Others may decide to take HRT for 10, 20 or more years as possible protection against **heart disease** or osteoporosis later in life. (See chapter 3 for more about these conditions.)

In short, the decision of whether to take HRT is not clear-cut. Most women find the issue complicated by the fact that there is no consensus in the medical field about the best uses of HRT. Research continues to evaluate the pros and cons. As new evidence comes to light, you and your medical practitioner can use these findings to make an informed choice for or against hormone replacement.

MENOPAUSE: NATURAL PATH OR DISEASE?

Q: From all the symptoms mentioned and the fact that many women undergo medical treatment for menopause, it sounds like menopause is a disease. Is it?

A: Good question—the answer to which depends on whom you talk to. Indeed, HRT raises issues about American health care in general. Are we treating menopause as a disease instead of as a natural stage in a woman's life? And if so, is that approach correct? Is the medical profession rushing to promote a therapy that may have unknown side effects 20 to 30 years down the road? Is it wise to tout HRT for all women when only certain women may need it?

The fact is that different doctors look at menopause differently—as do women. Some view menopause as a natural passage or natural stage in biological development. These doctors may believe that HRT is unnecessary or that it's useful for some women in certain situations, such as women at high risk for osteoporosis or women who had hysterectomies at young ages and prematurely lost the ability to produce estrogen.

Q: Are you saying that other doctors recommend HRT because they believe menopause is a disease?

A: Some doctors view menopause as a disease, an organ failure, a deficiency or a syndrome. They believe menopause must be medically treated in all women. A practitioner with this attitude will see HRT as beneficial to all women nearing menopause because all women are presumed "at risk." Still other doctors combine therapies.

Q: In that view, then, is menopause an "unnatural state"?

A: Closely related to the view that menopause is a disease is the idea that the postmenopausal state is unnatural. According to this argument, the female body was not designed to last many years past menopause. Today, however, women can live 30 or more years after menopause. This extended life span without estrogen is unnatural, according to the theory. Thus, it is unfair to deprive women of HRT and the benefits that it can produce. Proponents of this theory believe that women should take HRT if they want to.

Q: Are you saying some doctors believe that HRT is a natural therapy?

A: Well, it depends on whom you talk to. Some doctors view HRT as a natural therapy. They believe that because estrogen is a substance normally produced in a premenopausal woman's body, supplementation with estrogen is appropriate, natural and, in most cases, safe. We examine HRT in more detail in chapters 3, 4 and 5.

Q: Back to my earlier question—what other ways are there to treat menopausal symptoms?

A: Relieving symptoms and decreasing the risk of certain diseases can be approached in several ways. Lifestyle changes, natural hormone replacement and drugs are some of the ways to handle the symptoms of menopause. These different methods are covered in this book. So let's move on to chapter 2, in which we discuss the roles of diet and nutrition, exercise and certain medications.

2 NONHORMONAL APPROACHES TO MENOPAUSAL SYMPTOMS AND CONDITIONS

Q: I'm getting some of the classic vasomotor and genitourinary symptoms of menopause. What can I do to relieve them?

A: You have several options: proper diet and nutrition, exercise, medication and hormone replacement therapy (HRT). As you may recall, HRT is a medical treatment designed to supplement and/or replace some of the hormones that are produced in diminishing amounts during and after menopause.

Q: How can HRT help my vasomotor symptoms?

A: As we detailed in chapter 1, vasomotor symptoms are attributed to the sudden drop in estrogen that occurs at the time of menopause. HRT remedies this sudden drop by replacing lost estrogen. As a result, HRT decreases the frequency and severity of hot flashes and other vasomotor symptoms better than any other product on the market. Estrogen not only blocks the physiologic changes that cause hot flashes but also enhances the hypothalamus gland's production of natural **opiates**—chemicals that cause sleep and help ease pain.

Q: What about HRT and my genitourinary symptoms?

A: As you know from chapter 1, genitourinary symptoms develop after estrogen levels have remained low for months or years. HRT helps reverse vaginal atrophy, leading to fewer episodes of vaginitis and painful intercourse. Although how HRT affects urinary symptoms isn't clear, most doctors claim that it works, based on experience with patients (known in medical lingo as clinical experience). In chapter 3, we talk more in depth about what HRT can do for you.

DIET AND NUTRITION

Q: I'm not sure that I want to use HRT to treat my menopausal symptoms. But I am concerned about those long-term conditions associated with menopause that you mentioned in chapter 1— osteoporosis and heart disease. What can diet do?

A: A sound diet—one that contains enough vitamins and minerals and a variety of wholesome foods—can help relieve vasomotor and genitourinary symptoms and can be beneficial in protecting against osteoporosis and heart disease.

Q: Can any specific foods or supplements do the job?

A: Before we answer that, let's talk for a minute about a healthy diet. The foods you eat affect the health of your bones and the health of your heart—particularly during the menopausal and postmenopausal years, when many women develop problems with their bones and arteries. (We have more to say about this in chapter 3.) Even for women who are on

HRT, a well-crafted nutritional plan, or diet, is a necessary partner to hormone replacement. Without enough calcium, for instance, the bones cannot remain strong, no matter how much estrogen a woman takes.

Q: **But don't some women choose a healthy eating plan as an alternative to hormone replacement therapy?**

A: Yes. These women reevaluate and revise their diets in their peri- and postmenopausal years with long-term health in mind. They ensure that they're getting enough vitamins and minerals and not overloading their systems with too much protein, fat, sugar, caffeine or alcohol. Then they combine this dietary focus with an exercise program that improves bone and heart health.

Q: **Generally speaking, then, what kind of diet is best?**

A: One tailored to your lifestyle and health conditions, of course. Here are a few ideas to consider.

First, reduce the amount of protein you eat. Protein inhibits the absorption of calcium and increases the amount of calcium that is eliminated from the body through urine. If you're interested in avoiding osteoporosis, you might reexamine the amount of red meat and other protein that you eat. According to Robert P. Heaney, M.D., writing in *Calcium and Common Sense,* a 120-pound woman should eat no more than 44 grams (g.) of protein a day, or about eight ounces of meat a day. For a vegetarian or meatless choice, consider one and one-quarter cups of soybeans. Other experts put the protein figure lower, estimating that most middle-aged women can get adequate protein from four ounces of lean meat a day. If you wish to get higher amounts of protein, you need to get additional calcium to counterbalance what protein causes you to lose.

Second, watch your intake of phosphorus. Around 900 milligrams (mg.) of phosphorus a day can help build strong bones. At 1,700 mg. or more a day, it can trigger calcium excretion from the bones, which may reduce bone mass and contribute to osteoporosis. Foods containing high amounts of phosphorus are carbonated beverages, red meat and foods processed with phosphorus additives.

Q: **I guess I should avoid junk foods, right?**

A: That's a good idea. Diets that contain a lot of processed foods (which are high in fat, sugar and salt), fat, sugar, caffeine and alcohol are associated with an increased incidence of osteoporosis. Plus, too much sugar or processed food can change the pH level in the vagina and lead to vaginal infections.

Q: **You mentioned the vegetarian equivalent of a meat source, which has me wondering—should I consider a vegetarian diet?**

A: Perhaps. Vegetarian and vegan (no animal products) diets are associated with a lower risk of osteoporosis, possibly because people on these diets tend to lose less bone mass than people on meat-and-potatoes fare.

The diets of menopausal women should include foods that are high in **phytoestrogens**, chemicals that the body converts to estrogen. Sometimes called **plant estrogens**—although they are not actually estrogen itself—phytoestrogens seem to have the ability to diminish menopausal discomforts. Although phytoestrogens offer only about 1/400th of a dose of pharmaceutically prepared estrogen, the cumulative effect of a diet of weak estrogenic foods may offer some protection against menopausal symptoms and possibly against osteoporosis and heart disease.

Q: Which foods contain phytoestrogens?

A: Phytoestrogens come in two main classes: **isoflavones** (found in soybeans and soy products, such as tofu and miso) and **lignans** (found mainly in flaxseed, whole grains and some fruits and vegetables). Lesser amounts of phytoestrogens are found in apples, brown rice, carrots, green beans, peas, potatoes, red beans, sesame seeds, whole wheat and rye.

Q: What amount of phytoestrogens should I eat?

A: To ease menopausal symptoms, advises Holly Atkinson, M.D., editor of *Health News,* slowly increase your intake of soy products and other phytoestrogens. Your goal should be to build to 25 to 45 mg. of phytoestrogens a day. (As a point of reference, consider that there are roughly 2 mg. of plant estrogens per gram of soy protein.) **Flavonoids** are also helpful.

Q: What are flavonoids?

A: Colorful and aromatic compounds, flavonoids (or **bioflavonoids**) are found in fruits. They are weak plant estrogens that help stabilize collagen, the protein that gives structure to skin, bone, cartilage and connective tissue. Flavonoids are found in blackberries, blueberries, cherries, raspberries and other deeply colored foods, as well as in citrus rinds.

Q: Are there any precautions to be aware of regarding phytoestrogens?

A: First, let us say that many herbs that have been used for centuries to relieve hot flashes and other menopause-related discomforts happen to be sources of plant estrogens. Some herbs, such as ginseng, are relatively potent phytoestrogens; others, such as red clover, are relatively weak. The question really comes down to this: If you use phyto-estrogenic herbs and eat phytoestrogenic foods, are you actually taking a form of HRT?

Some doctors say yes, arguing that natural estrogen is still estrogen and can have the same positive—and negative— effects as HRT. But other practitioners point out that phyto-estrogens are considerably weaker than the estrogen in hormone supplements. Moreover, Michael Murray, N.D., and Joseph Pizzorno, N.D., writing in the *Encyclopedia of Natural Medicine,* point out that phytoestrogens tend to balance estrogen levels in the body.

If you're considering taking plant estrogens to relieve meno-pausal discomforts, be sure to discuss it with your practitioner. It's especially important to talk with your doctor if you have been advised not to take estrogen (perhaps you have a history of estrogen-dependent cancer) or if you have any other **contraindications** for HRT (see chapter 5).

Q: Let's get back to specific foods and supplements that can help menopausal symptoms, especially vasomotor ones. What should I know?

A: Let's start with vitamin E. Some experts believe that vitamin E can relieve hot flashes and other vasomotor symptoms. Good food sources of vitamin E include whole grains and cereals, nuts, and wheat germ and safflower oils.

But it's nearly impossible to get the recommended amounts from dietary sources; most women also need to take supple-ments. Taken in amounts of 400 international units (I.U.) several times a day (for a total of 800 to 1,600 I.U.), vitamin E can decrease the severity and frequency of symptoms in some women.

Vitamin E vaginal creams are also available to combat the problems of **atrophic vaginitis** (the shrinkage of vaginal tissue after menopause that can make sexual intercourse uncomfortable and lead to vaginal infections). These creams are often more effective than vaginal lubricants and perhaps as effective as the vaginal moisturizer Replens, according to studies.

Q: **Speaking of vitamins, are there any others that can help relieve menopausal symptoms and other menopause-related problems?**

A: Some women also report that the B vitamins and vitamin C can take the edge off menopausal discomforts, although there is no medical consensus on whether this really works. A practitioner who believes that these nutrients help reduce menopausal discomforts may recommend a B-complex vitamin supplement and an ideal dosage of vitamin C (often between 500 and 1,000 mg. a day).

Further, since low levels of the B vitamins and vitamin C are common in elderly people, some scientists believe that these deficiencies may play roles in the development of osteoporosis.

Osteoporosis and Diet and Nutrition

Q: **Osteoporosis is coming up a lot in this discussion. Can you tell me about it?**

A: Osteoporosis is a condition in which bones gradually lose their mineral content, becoming porous, thin and fragile. Osteoporosis causes pain, bone fractures (breaks) and loss of stature in its advanced stages. While not specifically a menopausal symptom, osteoporosis is a significant health hazard associated with menopause.

Q: How can I know if I'm at risk of osteoporosis?

A: Over the years, researchers have found that certain factors indicate a tendency to develop osteoporosis.

- Caucasian (particularly with a northern European heritage) or Asian race

- Slender or petite body frame

- Mother or father with **osteopenia** (low bone mass, a precursor of osteoporosis) or osteoporosis

- Primary residence in the northern areas of the country. More cases of osteoporosis occur among women in temperate climates than among women in the tropics.

- Premature menopause or early surgical menopause not followed by a regimen of hormone replacement

- History of irregular menstrual cycles

- History of **amenorrhea** (abnormal cessation of menstrual cycles)

- Late onset of menstruation (after age 16)

- Diet low in calcium

- Cigarette smoking

- Excessive caffeine or alcohol intake

- Lack of exercise

- Use of certain medications, such as steroids, anti-inflammatory drugs, **sedatives** and thyroid hormones

Q: How can specific dietary factors reduce the risk of or prevent osteoporosis?

A: Aside from the dietary factors we've already mentioned, including the B vitamins and vitamin C, other foods and supplements can make your bones strong. The minerals calcium and magnesium and vitamins D and K all play important roles in reducing the risk of or preventing osteoporosis.

Q: **I always hear that calcium is important to bones. In what way is it helpful?**

A: Representing about 40 percent of all the minerals found in your bones, calcium is responsible for bone strength. Your body also uses calcium to maintain brain function, aid in muscle contraction and assist in blood clotting. If you don't take in enough calcium in your daily diet, your body begins to siphon from your bones the calcium that it needs to do its other jobs. This can lead to **bone resorption**, the process by which bones dissolve and lose calcium. Bone resorption is common, too, in inactive people.

Q: **How much calcium do I need to take?**

A: Nutritionists say that most American women get only 500 to 700 mg. of calcium a day—not enough to prevent bone resorption. According to the National Institutes of Health, postmenopausal women should consume 1,500 mg. of calcium every day if they are not using HRT or 1,000 mg. every day in conjunction with HRT. And the Institute of Medicine says that women at risk of osteoporosis should consume between 1,000 and 1,300 mg. of calcium every day.

Q: **What is the best way to get calcium?**

A: The preferred approach is through dietary sources. Drinking three to four cups of milk a day (at 350 mg. of calcium per cup) is one way to get enough of the mineral. Eating calcium-rich foods is another. Such foods include one cup of cooked collard greens, eight canned sardines, one cup of calcium-fortified orange juice and one cup of yogurt (regular or low-fat), all of which contain at least 300 mg. of calcium. Lesser amounts of calcium are found in average servings of foods such as tahini, canned salmon (with bones) and cooked broccoli.

Q: If I don't eat any of the foods rich in calcium, can I take a supplement?

A: Yes. Taking a calcium supplement is another way to make sure you have enough calcium. Calcium is best absorbed in doses of 500 mg. or less, taken with a full eight-ounce glass of water. The supplement is best taken—in the sense of most efficiently absorbed—30 to 60 minutes after meals, unless otherwise noted by your practitioner.

Q: Which kind of calcium supplement should I take?

A: While calcium carbonate yields more calcium per pill, calcium citrate and calcium malate are more easily absorbed than calcium carbonate. According to Harris McIlwain, M.D., and Debra Fulghum Bruce, authors of *The Osteoporosis Cure,* many researchers agree that calcium citrate is about 60 percent more absorbable in the body, which means that your body can use more of what you take in.

Q: It sounds like the issue of calcium absorption is an important one. Do any other factors or substances inhibit it?

A: Yes. Inactivity, illness, some medications, caffeine, some foods and cigarette smoking can impede (but not necessarily stop) calcium absorption. Ask your doctor or nutritionist if you need to take more calcium to compensate for such factors.

Exercise and estrogen enhance absorption, which we talk about later in this chapter. In addition, remember to take adequate amounts of vitamins D, K and C and the mineral magnesium to ensure calcium absorption.

Q: Let's move on. What about vitamin D?

A: The right amount of vitamin D helps your body absorb calcium. About 400 I.U. per day is the recommendation of a number of experts. Sick adults and adults over the age of 65 need 800 to 1,000 I.U. daily. Too much vitamin D (more than 1,000 I.U. per day, according to some experts), though, can cause bone loss.

Q: What are the sources of vitamin D?

A: You can get vitamin D from being in the sun or from your diet. Women who are active outdoors may get enough vitamin D from sunlight, but as they age, the amount of vitamin D in the blood decreases by nearly 50 percent—the side effects of an age-related deficiency of an enzyme produced by the kidneys.

Q: What does sunlight have to do with vitamin D?

A: Sunlight helps your body manufacture natural vitamin D. Somewhere between 15 and 60 minutes of sunlight on your skin is needed for your daily dose. In general, women in northern climates need more exposure, and women in southern climates need less exposure. The exact amount is impossible to gauge.

Q: Which foods are rich in vitamin D?

A: Dietary sources of vitamin D include fatty fish (halibut, mackerel and salmon), vitamin D-enriched milk, liver, butter and egg yolks. You can also take a vitamin D supplement. Ask your doctor for a recommendation.

Q: Earlier you mentioned magnesium. How is it related to osteoporosis and the absorption of calcium?

A: Calcium and vitamin D work in concert with magnesium. Found in bone tissue, magnesium plays a role in bone formation and muscle contraction. The proper amount of magnesium helps your body use vitamin D to build strong bones.

Q: How much magnesium do I need?

A: The recommended ratio of calcium to magnesium is 2:1. For example, if you take 1,500 mg. of calcium, you need approximately 750 mg. of magnesium. This ratio is true for women in pre-, peri- and postmenopausal years. Many calcium supplements come with magnesium added in the proper amounts.

Q: Which foods contain magnesium?

A: Dark green vegetables, shellfish, legumes, cereals and nuts.

Q: What can you tell me about vitamin K relative to bone health?

A: Vitamin K helps keep calcium in the bones. Without vitamin K, bones can't mineralize, or form. This vitamin is abundant in leafy green vegetables. For those who don't eat their greens, fat-soluble chlorophyll capsules (available in health food stores) are another source. You don't need a lot of vitamin K to keep your bones healthy, so supplements are rarely necessary.

Heart Disease and Diet and Nutrition

Q: I think I get the picture. While certain vitamins and, in general, a healthy diet may help alleviate menopausal symptoms, a sound nutritional plan can have a significant impact on bone health. But earlier you said that diet and nutrition also play vital roles in preventing heart disease. Can we talk about that?

A: Yes. But first, let's define what we mean by heart disease. Cardiovascular disease—or heart disease, as it's often called—is a structural or functional abnormality of the heart or the blood vessels of the heart that impairs normal functioning. Heart disease is the leading cause of death among American women. According to the American Heart Association, more than one in five women has some form of cardiovascular disease. Although heart disease is much more common in men than in women before age 55, this difference begins to erode in women age 55 and older. By the time women reach their 80s, they have the same incidence of heart disease as men.

Q: How can I know if I'm at risk of heart disease?

A: Menopause itself is presented as a heart disease risk. And the more years you live postmenopausally without protective premenopausal levels of estrogen in your body, the greater the risk becomes. Whatever the precise mechanism of estrogen on heart disease, scientists assert that one thing holds true: When ovarian estrogen levels decline after menopause, women lose their protective edge and gradually develop the same risk of cardiovascular disease that men face.

But menopause isn't the only risk for heart disease. Additional factors are at play.

- A parent who had a heart attack before age 55. If this is true for you, your risk of heart attack may be four to five times greater than average, say Sheldon H. Cherry, M.D., and Carolyn D. Runowicz, M.D., in *The Menopause Book.*

- **Atherosclerosis**, the buildup of fatty deposits on the walls of the arteries

- High blood pressure, with readings above 140/90 mm Hg (millimeters of mercury) over a period of time

- Low levels of HDL (high-density lipoprotein), the "good" cholesterol, and/or high levels of LDL (low-density lipoprotein), the "bad" cholesterol. Cholesterol is a fatlike substance found naturally in animal foods such as meat, fish, poultry, whole-milk dairy products and egg yolks. Excess cholesterol causes fatty deposits to form along the walls of your arteries, which can lead to heart disease. We talk more about this in chapter 3.

- High triglyceride levels combined with low HDL cholesterol levels. Recent studies also show that triglycerides may have an impact on heart disease all by themselves. Like cholesterol, triglycerides are fats, or **lipids**. But they have a different chemical structure than cholesterol. Triglycerides, found in animal fats and plant oils, provide fats that your body uses for energy or places in its fat stores for later use.

- Smoking

- Diabetes, which can increase your risk of heart disease if it's not under control

- Overweight. In particular, people who collect fat around the waist are at higher risk of heart disease than people who accumulate fat around the hips.

- Sedentary lifestyle

- Stress

No one disputes the importance of the above risk factors in predicting heart disease. But there is debate over whether menopause puts *all* women at risk of heart disease or whether other risk factors must be present, too.

Q: How can diet and nutrition reduce the risk of or prevent heart disease?

A: Remember that a high-fat diet has been linked to heart disease, as well as to cancer and other diseases. Incorporating fiber, soy, certain antioxidants, and vitamins B_6 and folate into a low-fat diet can help guard against heart disease.

Q: How much fiber do I need?

A: Most fiber-rich foods have soluble fiber, which has been shown to lower cholesterol. According to the American Dietetic Association, most Americans eat only about 11 g. of fiber daily, while health experts recommend a minimum of 20 to 30 g. of fiber daily. Eat six servings of the following sources of soluble fiber daily to get 25 g. of fiber: a medium apple, a medium potato with skin, one-half cup of cooked beans, one cup of cooked brown rice or oatmeal or one-half cup of whole-grain cereal.

Q: Did you say soy may be helpful in protecting against heart disease?

A: Yes. New research from the University of Kentucky suggests that soy may lower a woman's chance of developing heart disease. Also, studies show that Asian women, who eat a soy-rich diet, have a lower incidence of cardiovascular disease, osteoporosis and hot flashes than American women.

Q: How much soy do I need to eat?

A: About 30 g. of soy protein daily is recommended to help fight heart disease. Good sources of soy protein include two cups of miso soup, one-half cup of "smoothie" made with soy powder, one and one-half cups of soy milk, three ounces of tofu, three ounces of tempeh and a three-ounce soy-vegetarian burger. Eat three of these foods daily to get 30 g. of soy protein.

Q: You said that antioxidants are also helpful against heart disease. What are antioxidants?

A: Substances that interfere with oxygen-generated, or oxidative, reactions. Antioxidants neutralize free radicals, unstable atomic or molecular fragments that can damage cells. Antioxidants believed to play roles in the prevention of heart disease are vitamins C and E, beta carotene and carotenoids. (Carotenoids are any of a group of red, yellow or orange pigments found in foods such as carrots, sweet potatoes and leafy green vegetables. The body converts these substances to vitamin A.)

Q: How are antioxidants related to heart disease?

A: Free radicals damage fat compounds in the body, causing the compounds to turn rancid and release more free radicals. This process, known as lipid peroxidation, is thought to trigger atherosclerosis, a key factor in cardiovascular disease. Antioxidants help in a process that stops these free radical chain reactions.

Q: How do I get antioxidants?

A: Through a diet rich in fruits and vegetables. Good sources include two medium raw tomatoes, one medium sweet potato, three and one-half ounces of strawberries, one cup of cooked spinach, two cups of romaine lettuce, one-half cup of red peppers, one ounce of peanuts, one cup of orange juice, one-half cup of carrots (raw or cooked), one-half cup of broccoli (raw or cooked) and one-half ounce of almonds. Eat five to nine servings daily.

Q: Can't I take a supplement?

A: Generally speaking, it's best to get your antioxidants from foods. Researchers know that certain carotenoids are very likely to be major players in reducing risk factors such as atherosclerosis. But their benefits may not be the same when carotenoids are isolated from one another in supplements or even when isolated from the other components of food that also promote cardiovascular health.

Q: OK. What about the other two vitamins that you mentioned, vitamin B$_6$ and folate? How are they related to heart disease?

A: Early research on this issue from Harvard University shows that women who consume at least 3 mg. of B$_6$ and 500 micrograms (mcg.) of folate every day are 45 percent less likely to develop heart disease than women who consume less than 1.1 mg. of B$_6$ and 200 mcg. of folate every day. The current Recommended Dietary Allowances (RDAs) of B$_6$ and folate for women are as follows: 1.3 mg. of B$_6$ between the ages of 19 and 50, 1.5 mg. of B$_6$ for women age 51 and older and 400 mcg. of folate.

EXERCISE

Q: What role does exercise play in relieving menopausal symptoms and preventing osteoporosis and heart disease?

A: Performed properly and regularly, exercise is one of the best measures for preventing long-term health problems. A carefully crafted program of exercise (and diet, as we've seen) can serve as an alternative or an addition to HRT, reducing the risk of osteoporosis and heart disease and even helping the body minimize the effects of hot flashes and other vasomotor changes during menopause. Indeed, exercise does something that HRT does not: It stimulates the formation of new bone. And possibly because exercise raises the brain levels of endorphins (natural body chemicals that reduce pain and enhance pleasure), many women find that regular exercise helps curb hot flashes or makes them less severe.

Q: Anything else?

A: Exercise also is very good for genitourinary symptoms and **urinary incontinence**—the tendency to leak urine, especially while laughing, sneezing or coughing. Urinary incontinence can be a problem for some women after menopause. Because estrogen levels are lower, the tissues of the vagina shrink, weaken and become dry, and the muscles around the bladder weaken. Any exercise that strengthens the back and stomach can tone the muscles that surround the bladder, urinary tract and vagina. Sexual intercourse (once or more a week) can keep the vaginal lining supple and the muscles surrounding the vagina and urethra firm.

Q: Whew! That's a big list of benefits of exercise. Now that it's on my mind—which exercises can help with urinary incontinence?

A: **Kegel exercises**, also known as **pubococcygeus exercises**, strengthen the pubococcygeus muscles— the band of tissue that extends from the pubic bone in the front of the abdomen to the last four vertebrae in the tailbone. Kegel exercises improve the ability to retain urine and strengthen the muscles of the vagina. In addition, Kegel exercises can increase circulation to the vagina, thereby improving lubrication.

Q: How are they done?

A: These simple exercises entail squeezing the muscles in the vaginal area, holding for several seconds, relaxing the muscles, then repeating. Practice the squeeze-hold-release-and-repeat pattern several times a day while standing, sitting or reclining.

To get the feel for doing Kegel exercises properly, practice during urination. Contract to stop the flow of urine midstream, then relax to release the flow.

Osteoporosis and Exercise

Q: Back to the issue of exercise and prevention of osteoporosis—what's the relationship between the two?

A: Exercise reduces the risk of osteoporosis by stopping or slowing bone loss. It also stimulates the formation of new bone. On the other hand, inactivity does not stress, or stimulate, bones. Consequently, they lose calcium.

Some studies have shown that exercise, combined with calcium supplementation, can increase bone mass and slow or prevent bone loss. One study showed that while a calcium-exercise routine is not as effective as an estrogen-exercise routine, the former had few side effects.

Q: When should I start exercising to prevent osteoporosis, and what are my options?

A: For protection against osteoporosis, exercise should be started at a young age and continued through life. But it's rarely too late to begin an exercise program, as long as you work with your medical practitioner before starting any new regimen. As a general rule, exercise should be moderately vigorous—enough to get you to work up a sweat but not so demanding that it stresses your body or causes injury.

As for how much, the general consensus is that an effective plan—one that maintains bone mass after menopause—entails at least 45 minutes of exercise per session, three to five sessions a week. Mix different types of exercise for variety and diverse benefits or as suggested by your medical practitioner or fitness expert.

You have several choices for exercise to help guard against osteoporosis: weight-bearing aerobic exercise; strength training; and balance, or appositive, exercise.

Q: Let's start with weight-bearing aerobic exercise. What is it, and how can it help?

A: Aerobic exercise is a steady activity that gets your heart pumping, conditions your body's muscles and makes you work up a sweat. Weight-bearing aerobic exercise is any form of exercise that stresses the bones and joints while working the cardiovascular system. Brisk walking, jogging, stair climbing, aerobic dancing, rope jumping, bicycling and cross-country skiing—all forms of weight-bearing aerobic exercise—performed for 20 to 30 minutes at a pace brisk enough to moderately raise your pulse rate are ideal options for most women.

Regular aerobic exercise strengthens the heart muscle. Make that aerobic exercise a weight-bearing exercise, and you can increase bone density—perhaps as much as 6 percent over two years.

Q: What about swimming?

A: Swimming is not considered a weight-bearing exercise because water buoyancy takes the weight off bones and joints. Thus, it doesn't stress bones and has no effect on bone density. But swimming is an excellent low-impact aerobic exercise, thanks to the buoyancy, which lowers the risk of impact-caused injuries such as fractures. Swimming is particularly good for orthopedic problems or for women coming late into an exercise regimen but still hoping to see the healthy effects of exercise.

Q: I'd like to supplement aerobic exercise with another form of exercise. What about strength training?

A: If prevention of osteoporosis is your goal, then aerobic exercise can certainly be alternated or combined with strength-training exercises for the upper body.

All the weight-bearing aerobic exercises mentioned earlier work to strengthen the muscles and bones of your lower body, but they don't build bones in your arms and torso. It's important to have healthy, dense bones in your back, for instance, to prevent a curved spine later in life. And strong arm bones also resist fractures in the wrists and forearms at any age.

Q: How does strength training build thicker, stronger bones?

A: It's all a matter of stress. When you stress your muscles with a carefully prepared plan of exercises, the resistance caused by the exercises forces your muscles to enlarge. At the same time that you're stressing your muscles, your muscles are pulling against your bones and stressing them. This stress, in turn, encourages your bones to grow, absorbing calcium and other minerals from the bloodstream and depositing the calcium and minerals inside the bones to form denser, thicker and stronger bone tissue. Thus, strength training results in stronger, calcium-rich bones—as long as your diet includes enough calcium for the bones to absorb, as we talked about earlier. In addition, muscles act as natural padding, and by strengthening them, your bones have more protection against fractures in case you would fall.

Q: Which exercises are good for strengthening the muscles?

A: Your choices include racquetball or tennis, swimming, energetic gardening (lifting and shoveling), modified push-ups, elastic resistance (using exercise bands), weight lifting with free weights, and weight-training machines.

Q: How much strength training is most effective?

A: Strength training is most effective when done two to three times a week throughout the entire year. Muscles need a 48-hour rest period after strength training to recuperate from the work you've put them through. Year-round training is needed to keep muscles and bones strong. Once you stop, your muscles and bones begin to lose strength.

Q: Can anyone at any age start strength training?

A: Yes. The key to muscle strengthening is to follow the right exercises and proceed at a proper rate (not too gradually and definitely not too quickly). Women with painful joints and women with advanced osteoporosis may be unable to launch into a weight-training program, for example, but age alone should not deter anyone from "pumping iron."

According to researchers at Pennsylvania State University, studies have shown that people in their 90s can triple their strength in less than two months when lifting weights. The training helps them resume everyday tasks such as household chores, which they were forced to stop due to the loss of strength brought on by years of inactivity.

In any event, check with your practitioner before starting a strength-training program, and work under the guidance of a trained instructor. Such expert advice is crucial with this type of exercise.

Q: What is balance exercise, and how can it help?

A: Balance, or appositive, exercise is a slow, concentrated movement that helps improve balance. Although balance exercise doesn't help any specific vasomotor or genitourinary symptom or directly prevent osteoporosis and heart disease, recent research suggests that slow, concentrated exercises can get circulation going and improve muscle tone and balance.

A study a few years back, reported in the *Journal of the American Medical Association*, found that elderly people who exercise are less likely to fall. Tai chi—a form of meditative exercise derived from a Chinese martial art—was the most beneficial form of exercise studied, reducing injuries caused by falls by 25 percent. Tai chi is a slow, graceful exercise that emphasizes good balance, making it a healthy option for women even in their 80s and 90s.

Yoga is another gentle exercise that can improve balance and increase muscle flexibility among women of all ages.

Heart Disease and Exercise

Q: What role does exercise play in heart disease?

A: Exercise reduces the risk of heart disease. Numerous studies have shown that an increase in physical activity not only benefits weight and levels of lipids (cholesterol and triglycerides) but also reduces stress, thereby taking care of the heart in many different ways at the same time.

Q: How much should I exercise to help prevent heart disease?

A: Most health experts recommend that exercise be performed three to five times a week and that each session last at least 20 minutes. And we've already talked about brisk walking, jogging, skipping rope and the like—weight-bearing aerobic exercises that help strengthen not only the bones but the heart, too.

Q: Is there anything more I need to know about exercise during the menopausal and postmenopausal years?

A: Just this: By combining several types of exercise, you can develop aerobic fitness (benefiting your health), muscular strength in your upper and lower body (improving balance) and greater bone density (making debilitating fractures less likely). Indeed, exercise is so effective that many doctors advocate a fitness plan for women who are on HRT. These doctors note that estrogen works better when a woman is active. And by combining exercise with calcium supplementation, you get additional protection against osteoporosis.

MEDICATIONS

Q: What kinds of medications relieve vasomotor and genitourinary symptoms?

A: As you know, HRT is often recommended to treat a number of vasomotor and genitourinary symptoms such as hot flashes, as well as long-term health problems such as heart disease and osteoporosis (see chapter 3). However, other drugs exist that can address menopausal discomforts and menopause-related health conditions. They are medications for hot flashes (progestin, **antihypertensives**, sedatives and **tranquilizers**); medications for vaginal dryness; and medications for osteoporosis (**salmon calcitonin, bisphosphonates, calcitriol, sodium fluoride** and **selective estrogen receptor modulators**, or **SERMs**).

Medications for Hot Flashes

Q: Start at the beginning—what about progestin?

A: Progestin—which can be either a natural or a synthetic form of progesterone—may be an option for women who want relief from hot flashes but who don't want to take estrogen. In this case, the physician will usually prescribe a low dose (2.5 mg. a day) of medroxyprogesterone acetate in pill form.

Another progestin, known as megestrol acetate, is used to relieve pain and other symptoms associated with advanced **breast cancer** and **endometrial cancer**. It can also help control hot flashes in women who have had cancer.

Q: Does progestin work for every woman?

A: No. Most mainstream medical practitioners believe estrogen is more effective in relieving hot flashes. When progestin does work, it starts providing relief in two to three weeks, with the best results achieved after a month or so of therapy. The higher the dose, the greater the relief. Higher doses, however, can lead to progestin-related side effects, such as **breakthrough bleeding**, water retention and bloating, breast swelling and tenderness, weight gain, depression and irritability.

Q: **I don't like the sound of that. Are there other drugs that can relieve hot flashes?**

A: Used to lower blood pressure, antihypertensives can also relieve hot flashes. While your doctor won't prescribe antihypertensive medication if your blood pressure is normal, these drugs are an option for menopausal women with elevated blood pressure (**hypertension**) who want relief from hot flashes.

One of these medications is clonidine (sold as Catapres, Catapres-TTS and Combipres and in generic form). It appears to reduce the frequency of menopausal symptoms by stabilizing the body's thermostat. Dry mouth and drowsiness are the drug's most common side effects. Constipation, weakness and insomnia are also reported side effects.

Methyldopa (sold as Aldomet, Aldoclor and Aldoril and in generic form) is another blood pressure medicine that reduces hot flashes. Side effects—which include dry mouth, headache, weakness and fatigue—are less common with this drug and generally start at the beginning of treatment.

Q: **You mentioned sedatives and tranquilizers. What can you tell me about them?**

A: Both sedatives and tranquilizers are prescribed, albeit infrequently, to relieve hot flashes. Sedatives decrease activity, relieve anxiety and calm a person. Tranquilizers also have a calming effect, lessening anxiety and tension and inducing drowsiness. Some tranquilizers can reduce muscle spasms.

Q: **Can you be more specific about how sedatives relieve hot flashes?**

A: They can have general, overall effects, or they can affect certain organs or systems, such as the vasomotor system—the part of the nervous system that controls the narrowing and widening of blood vessels. Sedatives relieve menopausal discomforts such as hot flashes and night sweats by selectively blocking the transmission of nerve impulses. One popular sedative for this purpose is Bellergal-S, an anti-spasmodic (a drug that prevents muscle spasms) used to treat palpitations, "nervous stomach" and vasomotor disturbances such as hot flashes, sweats, restlessness and insomnia. The drug's side effects—including dry mouth, constipation, tingling in the hands and feet and blurred vision—rarely occur, according to the *Physicians' Desk Reference*. However, it contains phenobarbital, a chemical that can be habit-forming.

Q: What about tranquilizers? They're used to calm, too, right?

A: Right. In a fashion similar to sedatives, the tranquilizers chlordiazepoxide (Librium) and diazepam (Valium) are sometimes prescribed to women who experience hot flashes, anxiety, irritability and mood swings during menopause. Librium reduces anxiety in ways scientists don't yet understand; Valium affects the hypothalamus—the part of the brain that controls the body's thermostat, as well as the endocrine system and parts of the nervous system. Because these drugs are addictive, they should be used for as short a time as possible. The *Physicians' Desk Reference* suggests less than four months.

Q: Are there other drawbacks to these medications?

A: Side effects can include drowsiness, weakness and fatigue. Also, withdrawal symptoms such as vomiting and cramping can occur if the drug is abruptly discontinued.

Medications for Vaginal Dryness

Q: What are the medications for vaginal dryness?

A: Vaginal lubricants are either prescription or non-prescription pharmaceutical products that counter vaginal dryness, which can lead to uncomfortable or painful sexual intercourse.

Q: Can you give examples of the types of lubricants available?

A: As we mentioned earlier, vitamin E vaginal creams are available to treat vaginal dryness.

Water-based lubricants (such as K-Y Jelly, Astroglide and Gyne-Moistrin Moisturizing Gel) and **vaginal suppositories** (Lubrin Vaginal Inserts Suppositories) soothe dry vaginal walls for several hours. They can be applied as often as needed, generally before intercourse. But be sure to check the manufacturer's directions.

Q: Is there anything I can get from my doctor for vaginal dryness?

A: Yes. **Vaginal estrogen cream** and vaginal estrogen suppositories—the latter made from finely ground estrogen—can be inserted or placed in the vagina to help keep the tissues of the vagina and bladder firm and to combat vaginal dryness and urinary tract infections. We have more to say about these estrogen-based products in chapter 4, when we discuss HRT.

Q: Is there anything that provides longer relief?

A: The moisturizing gel Replens reportedly gives longer relief, as each application lasts two to three days. Replens contains the chemical compound polycarbophil, which lowers vaginal pH to healthy levels, thus reducing the chance of vaginal infection. Replens can be applied before intercourse, but the optimum treatment plan is to use the gel two to three times a week—regardless of sexual activity—to keep the vagina healthy.

Again, where such products are concerned, check the manufacturer's directions for dosage and duration of efficacy.

Medications for Osteoporosis

Q: Are there medications to prevent osteoporosis?

A: Yes. Remember that we mentioned several: salmon calcitonin, bisphosphonates, calcitriol, sodium fluoride and SERMs. Let's start with salmon calcitonin, which is commonly called **calcitonin** and sold under the brand names Calcimar and Miacalcin (available as an injection and nasal spray). Calcitonin, a type of hormone that stimulates bone production, is approved by the Food and Drug Administration (FDA) to prevent further bone loss in postmenopausal women who already have osteoporosis. Calcitonin helps strengthen bone by steering calcium into it and slows bone resorption, which is the body's process of removing calcium from bones. Calcitonin also apparently decreases pain caused by vertebral fractures from osteoporosis.

Q: Does calcitonin have any side effects?

A: Possible side effects include allergic reactions, headache, dizziness, increased frequency of urination and abnormal fluid accumulation. Nasal irritation—including dryness, redness, itching and bleeding—is the most commonly reported side effect of Miacalcin Nasal Spray.

Any woman with an allergy to salmon should have an allergy test done before taking salmon calcitonin for the first time. In some cases, it can cause a severe, life-threatening allergic reaction.

Q: Is there anything else to know about calcitonin?

A: A woman should make sure that she has adequate calcium and vitamin D intakes while on calcitonin to prevent progressive bone loss.

Q: You mentioned bisphosphonates. What are they?

A: Bisphosphonates are a class of drugs that can prevent further bone loss. However, except for alendronate sodium (Fosamax), bisphosphonates are not approved by the FDA for this use. (Bisphosphonates are used to treat bone cancer and other bone-related conditions.) They work by reducing bone resorption.

Q: What does Fosamax do?

A: According to the manufacturer, 5 mg. of Fosamax daily prevents osteoporosis in postmenopausal women.

Results after two years of the ongoing six-year Early Post-menopausal Interventional Cohort (EPIC) study showed that treatment with Fosamax stopped bone loss in most women. Women treated with the drug significantly increased bone mass at the lumbar spine and hips by about 3.5 and 1.9 percent, respectively.

The FDA approved Fosamax for the *treatment* of osteoporosis in postmenopausal women in September 1995. Some years later—April 1997, to be exact—the FDA approved the drug for the *prevention* of osteoporosis in postmenopausal women and the *prevention* of fractures in postmenopausal women who already have osteoporosis.

Q: **This drug sounds promising. Are there any drawbacks?**

A: Yes. Fosamax carries very specific directions for administration: when to take it (time of day and proximity to mealtimes), what fluid to take it with and how much, and what protocol to observe after taking it. If these directions are not followed, upper-gastrointestinal problems can result. For best results, women should take Fosamax 30 minutes before breakfast (on an empty stomach) and avoid lying down afterward.

In addition, women with abnormalities of the esophagus, low levels of calcium in their blood or severe kidney disease or anyone unable to sit or stand upright for at least 30 minutes should not take Fosamax. Other side effects may include irritation and inflammation or ulceration of the esophagus.

Q: **What are some other bisphosphonates?**

A: Etidronate (Didronel) and pamidronate (Aredia) are two bisphosphonates that are injected into the body. Etidronate is also available in pill form and appears to prevent and treat osteoporosis of the spine. According to studies, pamidronate is effective in the treatment of postmenopausal osteoporosis and can increase bone mass and significantly reduce the frequency of new vertebral fractures. Again, though, these are drugs that have yet to be approved by the FDA specifically for the prevention and treatment of osteoporosis. They are approved for the treatment of other bone disorders. However, your doctor can prescribe them "off label," which means these drugs are used to prevent and treat osteoporosis even though they haven't yet been approved by the FDA for this purpose.

Q: Are there any other bisphosphonates?

A: Yes. **Risedronate** (Actonel) was approved by the FDA in March 1998 for the treatment of Paget's disease, but it has not been approved specifically for the prevention and treatment of osteoporosis. However, early research shows that this drug may help prevent osteoporosis and increase bone mass in early postmenopausal women. Research is ongoing.

Q: Earlier you mentioned calcitriol. What is it?

A: Calcitriol (Rocaltrol) is a potent form of vitamin D and a regulator of calcium. It appears to be an effective medication for osteoporosis, at least according to preliminary studies. Writing in *The Osteoporosis Handbook,* Sydney Lou Bonnick, M.D., says, "Studies have demonstrated that calcitriol can increase calcium absorption and increase the bone mass in the spine and forearm."

Q: What does sodium fluoride do for osteoporosis?

A: Once a mainstay of treatment for advanced osteoporosis and widely used for more than 30 years, this drug has fallen out of favor in the United States. Studies suggest that while sodium fluoride increases bone density in women who take it, it doesn't reduce the number of fractures.

However, new attention is being focused on this drug. A slow-release sodium fluoride, developed by researchers at the University of Texas Southwestern Medical School at Dallas, is awaiting approval by the FDA for the treatment of osteoporosis. A study published in the *Annals of Internal Medicine* found that women who combine slow-release sodium fluoride with calcium citrate supplements gain bone density in the spine and reduce their risk of future spine fractures.

Q: Are there any other medications to prevent osteoporosis?

A: In December 1997, the FDA approved a new drug, **raloxifene** (Evista), that helps protect the bones and possibly the heart. But it's important to note here that "there's not yet any evidence that raloxifene actually reduces the risk of fracture or heart attack," according to the May 1998 *Consumer Reports on Health*. For one thing, raloxifene doesn't have estrogen's ability to raise the level of "good" (HDL) cholesterol in the body (see chapter 3), although it may produce comparable reductions in the level of "bad" (LDL) cholesterol. And raloxifene doesn't relieve menopausal symptoms.

Q: Back to osteoporosis and raloxifene—what's the relationship between them?

A: First, let us say that raloxifene belongs to the new class of drugs known as SERMs. Also called a designer estrogen, raloxifene has the selective ability to act on many of the organs that estrogen does, but not the uterus and the breasts. Raloxifene doesn't cause the monthly bleeding or breast tenderness associated with estrogen replacement, and early data suggest that raloxifene doesn't increase the risk of uterine or breast cancer.

Raloxifene acts like estrogen on the bones by building bone density. But it seems to prevent bone loss less effectively than estrogen does, according to various reports. The drug's manufacturer, Eli Lilly, says raloxifene maintains bone and keeps it strong in most women. It is not known if raloxifene prevents fractures, however.

Q: What are some possible side effects?

A: Raloxifene may worsen some menopausal symptoms. Women who take raloxifene have a higher incidence of hot flashes and leg cramps than women taking estrogen. Like estrogen, raloxifene may increase the risk of developing blood clots in the lungs and legs. Long-term risks are unknown.

Nevertheless, raloxifene may prove useful for a woman who shouldn't go on estrogen replacement therapy but who still wants some protection for her bones and possibly for her heart. A final note: At about $65 per month, this new drug costs roughly twice as much as estrogen replacement therapy.

Medications for Heart Disease

Q: Are there medications to treat heart disease?

A: Actually, there are many medications available to treat heart disease, including nitroglycerin, diuretics, beta blockers, calcium-channel blockers and vasodilators, just to name a few. Because heart disease is a vast subject and beyond the scope of this book, it's best to research what's available on your own and discuss the different types of medications with your doctor. However, we discuss HRT and heart disease in the next chapter.

Q: Before we move on, I'd like to know one thing—is nonhormonal medication for the treatment of menopausal symptoms for me?

A: You should discuss this extensively with your physician. Your medical history, your views on HRT and your long-term health goals are all factors that will influence your decision. A combination of HRT, calcium supplements and exercise is the generally accepted approach for the prevention of osteoporosis, according to the American College of Obstetricians and Gynecologists. But before you decide, let's explore HRT in depth in the next chapter.

3 HORMONE REPLACEMENT THERAPY FOR MENOPAUSE AND BEYOND

Q: Now I understand how diet and nutrition, exercise and medications can help ease menopausal symptoms and also help prevent conditions that may occur after menopause. Can you briefly explain again what hormone replacement therapy does?

A: As you'll recall from chapters 1 and 2, hormone replacement therapy (HRT) is a medical treatment designed to supplement and/or replace the hormones estrogen and progesterone, which are produced in diminishing amounts during and after menopause. As we said in chapter 1, HRT is also known by several other names: estrogen therapy (ET), estrogen replacement therapy (ERT) and combined hormone therapy (CHT) or combination therapy. For the purposes of our discussion here, we may use these terms interchangeably—but always with the understanding that a woman who still has a uterus will be advised by her practitioner that one form of HRT, **unopposed estrogen** (estrogen alone, without another hormone), puts her at risk for endometrial cancer.

HRT can be used to treat both vasomotor and genitourinary menopausal symptoms, as well as to help prevent the long-term conditions associated with menopause. But before we talk further about the role HRT plays in these issues, let's take a brief look at its history.

HISTORY OF HRT

Q: OK. When was HRT first used?

A: Researchers first isolated estrogen and progesterone in the 1920s, and by the 1930s, synthetic forms of these hormones were produced for use during menopause. But it wasn't until the 1960s, when researchers understood the use of estrogen and progesterone as **oral contraceptives**, that HRT, in the form of estrogen therapy, became part of the medical arsenal.

Q: Wait a minute—which came first? Oral contraceptives or HRT?

A: Actually, the contraceptive pill came on the market first. It was followed by estrogen therapy. In the 1960s and early 1970s, many physicians encouraged their patients to begin daily doses of estrogen long before menopause and continue large doses for life. This form of HRT consisted of a synthetic estrogen called ethinyl estradiol and was given in less potent doses than oral contraceptives. Estrogen was portrayed as a miracle drug that could keep a woman young forever. Little thought was given to its long-term side effects.

Q: Was estrogen used only by menopausal women and by women seeking to prevent pregnancy?

A: No. From the 1940s to the early 1970s, doctors also widely prescribed another synthetic estrogen, diethylstilbestrol (DES), to reduce the risk of miscarriage. In 1971, a link was found between the use of DES during pregnancy and a rare form of vaginal cancer. That year, the Food and Drug Administration withdrew its approval of DES for use as a pregnancy medication.

Q: Were there any other revelations about estrogen at that time?

A: Yes. Even more evidence about estrogen's drawbacks was made public in the 1970s. Researchers disclosed that women who had been using the contraceptive pill since their 20s and 30s faced a much greater risk of heart attack in their 40s, especially if they were smokers. And in 1975, estrogen therapy for menopause was linked to dramatically increased rates of cancer of the uterus—in the range of four to 14 times the norm, depending upon how long a woman had taken the hormone and at what strength.

Q: Did women stop using estrogen? And how did the medical industry respond?

A: First things first. Yes, as these disturbing figures came to light, prescriptions for estrogen therapy plummeted from 1975 to the mid-1980s. The medical world and the pharmaceutical industry scrambled to adjust. DES was removed from the market. Doses of estrogen were reduced for both oral contraceptives and HRT. In addition, researchers developed a new so-called natural conjugated (combined) estrogen that was collected from animals and that more closely matched the chemical composition of human estrogen.

Finally, to address the problem of endometrial cancer, doctors began prescribing progestin in addition to estrogen. The result was combined hormone therapy—which today is the mainstay of HRT.

Q: Why was progestin added?

A: Scientists discovered that unopposed estrogen stimulates the growth of cells in the uterus. Without progesterone to cause a menstrual period and thus shed those cells, the lining of the uterus (endometrium) becomes too thick, setting the stage for a slow-growing form of cancer.

Q: Am I right in saying that HRT is popular once again?

A: Yes, as far as the top 10 pharmaceutical sales "hit parade" is concerned. Today, the most commonly prescribed drug in the United States is Premarin, a conjugated estrogen.

HRT AND MENOPAUSAL SYMPTOMS

Q: Let's move on. I know the decision to use HRT is an individual one, but as far as the medical world is concerned, what will HRT achieve?

A: There are persuasive reasons to use HRT beginning at the time of menopause. They include the following:

- To combat menopausal symptoms such as hot flashes
- To combat atrophy (shrinking of tissues)
- To combat loss of bone mass
- To protect against heart disease

Remember, though, that for most women, these benefits are not achieved without some adverse effects. These might be minor but bothersome problems such as breast tenderness, migraines, leg cramps, nausea and vomiting. Or HRT's possible adverse effects may be serious, even life-threatening. We talk about these issues in chapters 4 and 5.

Q: How well does HRT help reduce vasomotor symptoms such as hot flashes?

A: Traditionally, the major reason for the use of HRT has been relief of menopausal symptoms. Only recently has there been a push to consider its potential benefits in preventing osteoporosis and heart disease. That said, the consensus in the medical community is that estrogen decreases the frequency and severity of hot flashes and other vasomotor symptoms better than any other product on the market. As you may recall from chapter 2, estrogen not only blocks the physiologic changes that cause hot flashes but also enhances the hypothalamus gland's production of chemicals that cause sleep and help ease pain.

"Estrogen therapy ameliorates these vasomotor symptoms in the majority of cases," write Bruce R. Carr, M.D., and Jean D. Wilson, M.D., in *Harrison's Principles of Internal Medicine*. You can expect to see marked improvement two weeks to two months after you start therapy.

Q: How can HRT help relieve sleep problems?

A: By relieving hot flashes, HRT can also help with sleep problems. As we said in chapter 1, women with frequent hot flashes may repeatedly awaken because they feel warm, even sweaty. Over the course of days and months, such disrupted sleep can cause memory lapses and feelings of anxiety. When the hot flashes are eliminated, sleep problems are less common.

Q: Can HRT help ease genitourinary symptoms, too?

A: Yes. For one, HRT helps combat atrophy—in this case, the degeneration of estrogen-sensitive tissues in the body. Genitourinary symptoms—including dryness, itchiness and a sensation of burning in the vagina—are reflections of atrophic changes in response to declining estrogen levels. Further, the vagina's pH rises, becoming more alkaline. The declining acidity level makes the vagina susceptible to inflammation and infection. At the same time, a woman may notice that her body is producing less vaginal lubrication during sex.

According to the May 1998 American College of Obstetricians and Gynecologists (ACOG) Educational Bulletin, "Use of systemic estrogen replacement or local estrogen creams and ...suppositories [see chapter 4] can reverse many if not all of these changes. Hormone replacement therapy can decrease the risk of urinary tract infection...."

Q: Can HRT help prevent other urinary symptoms?

A: Hormone replacement's effect on urinary symptoms such as incontinence and nocturia is less clear. Most doctors claim that it works, based on experience with patients (known in medical lingo as clinical experience). An analysis of 23 studies evaluating the effectiveness of HRT in treating urinary incontinence, published in *Obstetrics and Gynecology* some years back, found only "subjective" improvements. The data "seem to support the impression of benefit of estrogen therapy" for urinary incontinence, the authors of the analysis write, and "no evidence was shown to contradict use." The ACOG Educational Bulletin notes that "the ring delivery system [vaginal administration of estrogen] has been shown to relieve vaginal and urinary symptoms without increasing systemic estradiol levels"—in other words, the effect is localized, usually restricted to the vagina, urethra and bladder. (See chapter 4 for discussion of the many forms of HRT.)

Q: What about the skin changes you mentioned in chapter 1? Can HRT help with them?

A: The answer is a very cautious yes. HRT is sometimes promoted as a medication to treat problems that are neither vasomotor nor genitourinary, such as sagging breasts and drier, looser skin. Although experts are unsure if estrogen prevents aging and wrinkling, they know it helps maintain a cushion of oil-producing collagen under the skin, making skin seem more flexible and younger. You see, some studies have shown that estrogen replacement increases the thickness and collagen content of the skin. (You probably remember that when estrogen levels decline, skin becomes thinner and loses some elasticity. It also loses some collagen, whose job is to act like a padding under the skin, making the skin more resilient.)

Truth is, though, some doctors extrapolate from this and say that estrogen will keep the skin looking youthful. Daniel R. Mishell Jr., M.D., writes in *Conn's Current Therapy, 1995,* "Systemic estrogen use can retard the wrinkling and thinning of the skin that occurs postmenopausally."

Without a doubt, however, this is a subject of some debate. A 1997 University of California, Los Angeles, study reported that HRT users developed fewer wrinkles than nonusers. But according to Susan M. Love, M.D., in *Dr. Susan Love's Hormone Book,* only a handful of scientific studies on estrogen and skin changes have been done, and they show little or no relationship between the two.

Q: So what's the bottom line?

A: The fact is, no studies have proven that estrogen use can undo the influence of other factors that age skin and reduce its elasticity—factors such as heredity, cigarette smoking, sun exposure, climate and overall health.

Q: Can HRT help alleviate the mood changes and depression often associated with menopause?

A: This is another controversial area. Irritability, anxiety, depression, memory lapses and inability to concentrate have all been blamed on menopause. The debate revolves around twin issues: How much of this is due to a lack of estrogen, and how much is due to other stresses in a woman's life? Possibly because of its effects on symptoms of menopause such as hot flashes and sleep disturbances, HRT may improve a woman's state of mind.

As previously mentioned, though, numerous studies have determined that in emotionally healthy women, menopause by itself does not cause depression. But experts do agree that having to cope with distressing symptoms may contribute to depression.

Q: **You said earlier that HRT can help prevent long-term postmenopausal conditions. What are you talking about?**

A: Osteoporosis and heart disease.

HRT AND OSTEOPOROSIS

Q: **I hear a lot about osteoporosis. Do many people have it?**

A: Ten million Americans—80 percent of whom are women—have osteoporosis, and another 18 million have low bone density that places them at increased risk of fractures, according to 1998 figures from the National Osteoporosis Foundation.

Q: **How does hormone replacement combat loss of bone mass and help protect against osteoporosis?**

A: When estrogen is absent from the bloodstream, some women begin to lose bone mass. Thus, bones become porous and brittle. In its advanced stages, osteoporosis causes pain, bone fractures and loss of stature—the so-called dowager's hump seen in many older women.

To answer your question simply, though: "Estrogen works to

prevent osteoporosis by stimulating cells in the bone to maintain their function to retain calcium and to maintain the actual structure of the bones, keeping them strong and thereby reducing the risk of breaking bones," says Graham A. Colditz, M.D., in *Scientific American Presents:Women's Health* (Summer 1998).

According to the May 1998 *Consumer Reports on Health,* "In a recent multicenter study...three years of estrogen replacement therapy boosted bone density by 5 percent in the spine and 2 percent in the hips, compared with a loss at both sites in the placebo [inactive pill] group." The article goes on to recount other research that suggests HRT also helps preserve bone in the jaw and, thus, helps women retain their teeth.

Estrogen also stimulates the thyroid gland's production of calcitonin (a hormone that stimulates bone production), and it may increase the body's ability to absorb calcium from the intestines.

Q: Are you saying that estrogen can rebuild bone?

A: No. However effective in stopping bone loss, estrogen cannot rebuild bone.

Q: Earlier you mentioned fractures associated with osteoporosis. Why are fractures a particular concern?

A: Fractures in the spine lead to stooped posture. Fractures in the wrists can be inconvenient; those in the hips can be incapacitating, necessitating surgery or prolonged care. In addition, fractures can be life-threatening, particularly in the elderly: Five to 20 percent of older men and women who have hip fractures die within 12 months of their injuries— often from complications of hip surgery—and 15 to 25 percent are permanently disabled, according to *Current Obstetric and Gynecologic Diagnosis and Treatment.* The projected health care costs for hip fractures alone is more than $7 billion a year, says the ACOG.

Q: It sounds like osteoporosis is a natural part of aging. Is it?

A: To varying degrees. An adult's bones are at their peak density around age 35. Bone mass slowly declines in women as well as men after age 40. Once a woman reaches menopause, however, the decline in bone mass continues at a much quicker pace. This accelerated phase lasts eight to 10 years, after which bone loss slows to the premenopausal rate. In general, women lose 50 percent of **trabecular bone** and 30 percent of **cortical bone** during their lives; men lose 30 percent of trabecular bone and 20 percent of cortical bone.

Q: Wait a minute—what's the difference between trabecular and cortical bone?

A: Your bones are made from a combination of two types of tissue: trabecular bone, a porous tissue; and cortical bone, a dense, hard tissue. Flat bones and the vertebrae (backbones) are primarily trabecular bone surrounded by a thin layer of cortical tissue. Long bones such as the femur (thighbone) are primarily cortical tissue.

Q: Is gradual bone loss a problem for all women?

A: If your bones are strong to begin with, the gradual loss of bone tissue may not pose a problem as you get older. If your bones are thin in your 30s, you run a greater risk of experiencing fractures in your life. If your bone density is 20 to 30 percent lower than average, you have osteopenia (low bone mass). If your measurement is more than 30 percent lower than average, you have osteoporosis. Bone loss in the range of 30 to 40 percent can lead to fractures in the spine and stooped posture.

Q: **I know we talked about the risk factors for osteoporosis in chapter 2. If one or more of these factors apply to me, will I get osteoporosis?**

A: Not necessarily. Nor does it mean you should automatically start HRT, although some doctors rely on these risk lists in recommending hormone therapy. A menopausal woman who is thought to be at risk should first be given an osteoporosis screening test—one or more diagnostic tests that include **photo absorptiometry scans** and **CT (computerized tomography) scans**.

Q: **How can a screening test tell if my bones are weak?**

A: The only clearly visible sign of bone loss is the dowager's hump, and by the time a woman has this curvature, she has lost up to 50 percent of the bone tissue in her vertebrae. On the other hand, bone density tests show what the naked eye cannot see. They provide a snapshot, so to speak, of current bone thickness.

Q: **Can you tell me more about what an osteoporosis screening test shows?**

A: Certainly. It can show how you compare with a statistically average woman. If your bone mass is 20 percent lower than the statistically average woman's bone mass, the doctor sees a cause for concern. If the results show *some* bone loss, but less than 20 percent, the case is less clear. In such a case, one test alone can't necessarily predict whether you're on the fast track to osteoporosis. Your doctor may want to perform another test in six months to a year to track changes in bone mass, estimate the rate of bone loss (remember—some bone loss is inevitable) and decide if steps need to be taken to slow the rate of loss.

In any event, a bone density test is most informative when compared against a baseline, which is the first test with which later ones are compared.

Q: When should this first test be performed?

A: In the context of bone health, the best baseline test would be one done in your mid- to late 30s, when your bones are at their strongest. But baseline bone density tests are not commonly administered that early in life. Instead, doctors often have to perform a series of bone density tests over several months or years to get an accurate picture of how quickly your bone mass is changing. Thus, if you're planning to take HRT solely to protect against the possibility of developing osteoporosis, you'd be wise to have your doctor order a bone density test before you begin therapy. Your bones may be strong and healthy, making hormone replacement unnecessary. In short, even though you may fit the "at risk" category, you may never develop osteoporosis.

Q: Briefly then—what specific tests measure bone mass?

A: Here are some of the most common.

- **Radiographic absorptiometry (RA).** This is basically an x-ray taken of the hand to determine bone density, detect fractures and help the medical practitioner diagnose osteoporosis. X-rays can't detect bone loss until 30 percent of bone mass has already disappeared. For this reason, x-rays are not the best method for diagnosing osteoporosis early.

- **Single-photon absorptiometry (SPA).** In this (an increasingly outmoded test), radioactive iodine is used to determine the bone density of the wrist or heel. The radiation dose is about one-tenth of the dose used in RA.

- **Dual-photon absorptiometry (DPA).** This test, also using radioactive iodine, measures the density of the spine, hip or thighbone. The radiation dose is less than the dose used in SPA.

- **Dual-energy x-ray absorptiometry (DEXA).** A DEXA scanner emits very low levels of x-ray radiation, and a detector measures the amount of radiation absorbed by bone. The more radiation absorbed, the denser the bone. This test can be done on any part of the body—wrist, arm, spine, hip or thighbone.

- **Quantitative computerized tomography (CT scan or QCT scan).** A CT scan can measure trabecular bone within the vertebrae, the area where compression fractures occur, and create a 3-D image of the spine. But it does so with a much higher dosage of radiation than DPA or DEXA.

To find a bone density testing center near you, ask your medical practitioner or call the National Osteoporosis Foundation at 800-464-6700.

Q: Should I take HRT to prevent osteoporosis?

A: We can't answer that—it's an issue for you and your practitioner to hash out. It's true that estrogen plays a crucial role in preserving bone tissue. If you are at high risk of osteoporosis, even diet and exercise may not be enough to halt bone deterioration. But if your bone density is normal, then HRT may not improve it any further. You could possibly do yourself some harm by taking HRT unnecessarily (see chapter 5).

HRT AND HEART DISEASE

Q: I know you mentioned it earlier, but what is heart disease?

A: Heart disease is a structural or functional abnormality of the heart or the blood vessels of the heart that impairs normal functioning. The American Heart Association says that in the United States, all cardiovascular diseases combined claim the lives of about 505,000 females annually, while all forms of cancer combined kill about 257,000 females annually—making heart disease, as we said earlier, the leading cause of death among American women.

Q: You said in chapter 2 that experts believe menopause puts women at risk of heart disease. Can we talk more about this?

A: Certainly. True, menopause itself is presented as a heart disease risk. But remember—it's not the only risk. (See the other risks listed on pages 48-49.) There is debate over whether menopause puts *all* women at risk of heart disease or whether other risk factors must be present, too. Kristen E. Smith, M.D., and Howard L. Judd, M.D., writing in *Current Obstetric and Gynecologic Diagnosis and Treatment,* report, "Studies have suggested that the protective effect of estrogens on the heart is greatest in women with known risk factors for heart disease."

According to the ACOG, many studies suggest that one of the mechanisms by which estrogen helps protect against heart disease is by lowering LDL (low-density lipoprotein), the "bad" cholesterol, and increasing HDL (high-density lipoprotein), the "good" cholesterol. In research conducted on animals, estrogen reduces the amount of fat (known as lipids) deposited on artery walls, decreases the amount of cholesterol deposited in blood vessels and increases blood flow. For these reasons, estrogen is thought to give women a protective edge, or advantage.

Q: But earlier you said the advantage erodes after women reach age 55, right?

A: We said that heart disease—which is more common in men than in women before age 55—plays catch-up in women the years after age 55. So by the time women reach their 80s, they have the same incidence of heart disease as men.

Q: So can HRT help prevent heart disease?

A: Most experts agree that supplemental estrogen gives some measure of protection to postmenopausal women who are susceptible to heart disease. In the Nurses' Health Study, a massive study of registered nurses begun in 1976 and continuing today, more than a decade of data has shown that those women taking estrogen are at significantly decreased risk of major coronary disease.

Q: Is there a benefit if a woman takes progesterone as well?

A: Good question. This is an issue that researchers have long wondered about—namely, whether the addition of progesterone might undercut HRT's benefits, largely because the combination raises HDL levels somewhat less than unopposed estrogen does. However, in the words of *Consumer Reports on Health,* "Recent research has shown that the two hormones lower LDL, fight hardening of the arteries and prevent [the harmful process of] oxidation just as effectively as isolated estrogen does." What's more, the combination therapy may reduce Lp(a), "an especially harmful cousin of LDL," more effectively.

In the Nurses' Health Study, researchers have found that women taking either regimen—unopposed estrogen or combination therapy—have roughly the same 50 percent drop in coronary deaths.

Q: So should I take HRT to protect against heart disease?

A: We can't answer that. Frankly, the answer depends on whether you and your doctor believe that you are at risk of heart disease.

You see, some doctors promote HRT as a package deal: By taking it, they say, you can minimize menopausal symptoms, reduce the risk of osteoporosis and reduce the risk of heart disease. Others prefer to recommend HRT only for women at high risk of heart disease—at least until all the data about estrogen have been brought in. "As it stands today, postmenopausal women should not be taking hormones as the sole method of preventing heart disease," say Sheldon H. Cherry, M.D., and Carolyn D. Runowicz, M.D., in *The Menopause Book.* "Women should take other steps to prevent heart disease, with or without hormone therapy."

However, the story may be different for older women who already have heart disease. In a recent study at Wake Forest University, researchers found that daily use of combination HRT did not decrease the incidence of death or heart attack among older women *who already had heart disease.*

HRT AND STROKE

Q: If HRT can help prevent heart disease, can it also prevent stroke?

A: Researchers are examining estrogen's role in preventing stroke—what doctors call a **cerebrovascular accident**. Stroke can cause weakness, temporary or permanent paralysis, and even death. Stroke is a major contributor to long-term disability and is the third leading cause of death among postmenopausal women in developed countries.

Q: What causes a stroke?

A: A blood clot that blocks a blood vessel or a hemorrhage (excessive bleeding) from a blood vessel in the brain.

Q: I read that women who have histories of abnormal blood clotting are generally told not to take HRT. Isn't it flying in the face of common sense to use hormones to reduce the risk of stroke?

A: You're right—it does seem so. And in chapter 5, we talk about this caveat for women with such histories. As for the sense of using hormones to reduce the risk of stroke, researchers do not yet have a definitive answer. Several studies have looked at the stroke-protective aspects of HRT, and the results have been conflicting. Clearly, then, more research needs to be done before HRT can be recommended as a preventive therapy for stroke. You should just be aware that medical science continues to search for more uses for HRT.

HRT AND OTHER CONDITIONS

Q: Speaking of research on more uses for HRT, didn't I read that HRT can help with Alzheimer's disease and other memory lapse disorders?

A: Yes. But let us caution that the evidence for other possible benefits is newer and less certain than the evidence for bone and heart protection. Such connections are being explored, but the findings are often inconclusive and the matter is one of some debate.

Because Alzheimer's—a progressive, degenerative brain disease that impairs memory, thinking and behavior—is more common in women than in men (men are more likely to develop other forms of dementia), scientists are considering a possible link to the hormone estrogen. "In theory," says *Consumer Reports on Health,* "estrogen may improve brain function by boosting levels of certain enzymes crucial to learning and memory, stimulating the growth of brain-cell connections and increasing cerebral blood flow."

In one recent study, a lower rate of Alzheimer's disease was found among women who took estrogen, compared with women who did not. This is one of several preliminary studies that show a possible link between estrogen and prevention of Alzheimer's disease. Studies have also found an improvement in cognitive function in elderly women who were diagnosed with Alzheimer's and who were placed on estrogen therapy.

Q: Seems like the link is pretty clear. Where's the debate?

A: Well, other researchers question the methods and results of such preliminary studies. An analysis, published in the March 4, 1998, *Journal of the American Medical Association,* of relevant medical literature from January 1966 through June 1997 looked at 10 studies that addressed the association between postmenopausal estrogen replacement therapy and the risk of Alzheimer's disease and other dementias. The researchers concluded, "There are plausible biological mechanisms by which estrogen [therapy] might lead to improved cognition, reduced risk for dementia or improvement in the severity of dementia." However, the authors say that such studies may not have not been conducted properly. Consequently, they recommend that large, placebo-controlled studies be conducted to determine if estrogen therapy can actually reduce the risk of developing Alzheimer's disease and other dementias. (By the way, this type of study— placebo-controlled, in which a group receiving an experimental treatment is compared with a so-called control group receiving a placebo, or inactive treatment—is often described as an optimal study design.)

Q: Are there any other benefits of long-term HRT?

A: Possibly. As more and more studies are done regarding HRT, some other potential benefits are coming to light.

Q: Like what?

A: According to the November 27, 1997, *Medical Tribune,* researchers at the University of East Anglia in Norwich, England, found that women are less susceptible to cataracts than men are before age 50. But after age 50, this trend reverses sharply. Writing in that issue of the *Medical Tribune,* the lead researcher says, "While the ability of both the male and female lens to cope with eye stress decreases with age, the rate of decline is much steeper in women." Postmenopausal women who take HRT may be able to avoid this, postulate the researchers.

Q: What else?

A: HRT may lower the risk of colorectal cancer in postmenopausal women. Again using data from the Nurses' Health Study, researchers found that the risk of colorectal cancer was 33 percent lower among women actively using HRT. This protection diminished among women who had stopped hormone therapy, and there was no protection for women who had not taken estrogen for five or more years.

In another study of more than 7,000 California women, estrogen replacement was tied to a reduction in the risk of colorectal cancer. Again, the protection afforded by estrogen was highest among current or recent users.

Q: Are there any other health problems or conditions that HRT may help?

A: Yes. A study conducted at the University of Manchester in England found that estrogen may speed wound healing in postmenopausal women. True, the study was small, and more research is needed before we reach definitive conclusions. Nonetheless, these results are interesting. The rates of wound healing in older women on HRT were similar to those of younger women; furthermore, the women on HRT had taken the hormones for as few as three months.

Q: Any other conditions?

A: Estrogen therapy may reduce both the incidence and the severity of type-2 diabetes (once known as adult-onset diabetes). This type of diabetes occurs when the body fails to use insulin properly and is more common among people who are over age 45 and who are overweight.

In studies presented in 1998 at the annual scientific session of the American Diabetes Association, researchers concluded that postmenopausal women on estrogen replacement therapy are less likely to develop type-2 diabetes and, if they already have the disease, are better able to maintain proper blood sugar levels.

CHOOSING PREVENTIVE HORMONE THERAPY

Q: Speaking of cancer, heart disease and stroke and even chronic diseases such as diabetes, I can't help but ask—will HRT increase my chances of living longer?

A: A study, published in the June 19, 1997, *New England Journal of Medicine,* found that on average, women who use postmenopausal hormones have a lower rate of mortality than nonusers—particularly for death due to coronary heart disease. However, the study also concluded that the "survival benefit diminishes with longer duration of use and is lower for women at low risk for coronary disease. . . . "

In this analysis of participants in the Nurses' Health Study, researchers found that "whereas lower rates of cardiovascular mortality were maintained for long-term users, the risk of breast cancer mortality in this [group] was elevated by 43 percent after 10 years of taking hormones. Thus, with additional years of use, expected [survival benefits] were, in part, offset by the risk of breast cancer. . . . "

Q: That sounds like a mixed blessing, depending upon the individual woman and how long she uses HRT. But what's this business about breast cancer?

A: We discuss the explosive issue of a possible link between estrogen and breast cancer, along with other conditions that may have a connection to estrogen, in chapter 5.

Q: Whew! Sounds like there are a lot issues to be thought over and discussed with my practitioner. What else could I possibly need to know?

A: First, let us say that HRT, as you've seen, can be taken to reduce menopausal symptoms or to possibly protect against osteoporosis or heart disease. And as we said before, many doctors even offer it as a package deal—one that can protect you against all those potential problems and risks. More skeptical physicians believe that only women at high risk of osteoporosis and heart disease should take these drugs. And most agree that HRT is not suited for all women.

The decision to take HRT is yours to make. And chapters 4 and 5 are designed to help you make that very personal decision. If you do decide to take long-term preventive hormone therapy, you'll be faced with several smaller but equally important choices. They include the following:

- *Deciding whether to take estrogen alone (unopposed estrogen) or in an estrogen/progestin combination.* Estrogen alone or in combination with progestin offers protection against heart disease. But as we've said before, unopposed estrogen is not recommended if you still have a uterus.

    If you choose combination therapy, you can select estrogen and progestin in a variety of formulations and cycles (see chapter 4).

- *Deciding when to begin therapy.* While hormone replacement can begin at any age during the menopausal process, most doctors suggest that you make your decision soon after menopause—or at the time that your periods cease. They advise that HRT can slow down the otherwise rapid decline in bone mass during the first decade after your last menstrual period. Further, HRT is thought to best protect against heart disease when taken early. But let us stress this: Not every expert is in total agreement with this strategy.

    Some doctors even recommend HRT during the perimenopausal years. To combat irregular and erratic periods, your doctor may recommend a weeklong regimen of progestin only, which will cause you to menstruate each month until your estrogen levels become too low. Or estrogen in combination with progestin may be recommended to fend off any menopausal discomforts you may be having in the perimenopausal years. Few doctors, however, recommend HRT for women who are still menstruating.

- *Ensuring you get adequate medical care.* Long-term hormone use requires a more diligent commitment to getting medical care. As with any drug, the longer you take hormones, the greater your chance of experiencing long-term side effects.

- *Deciding how long to take hormones.* Most HRT proponents believe that once you start preventive therapy, you can (and should) take it for life to maintain its protective benefits. The more conservative approach points out that you don't have to take it forever.

In fact, a substantial number of women who are prescribed hormone therapy "either do not fill the prescription or discontinue the therapy within less than five years because of perceived cancer risks (principally breast cancer) or adverse side effects," says the ACOG. This, according to the venerable group of obstetricians and gynecologists, points to the absolute need for woman and practitioner to coordinate strategies regarding the benefits and adverse effects of estrogen replacement therapy.

Q: What kinds of side effects are there?

A: Short-term side effects of HRT include breast tenderness, migraines, leg cramps, nausea and vomiting. In addition, HRT's possible long-term adverse effects may be serious, even life-threatening. (See chapters 4 and 5.)

Q: Did you say the adverse effects could be serious or even life-threatening?

A: Yes. We have said time and again that one form of hormone therapy, known as unopposed estrogen therapy, increases the risk of endometrial cancer two- to 15-fold.

Several recent studies suggest that estrogen therapy increases the risk of gallstones two- to threefold. Another potential effect of HRT is how it affects a woman's risk of breast cancer. More than 50 studies have been conducted over the past 25 years to address this question, and researchers dispute the findings. Some say the data show no connection between HRT and breast cancer; others read into the data an overall increased risk related to dosage and duration of use. For some women, the chance of risk—no matter how small— is enough to make them question the value of HRT.

But before we explore these controversies and issues, let's move to chapter 4, where we discuss what forms HRT comes in, how much to take and for how long.

4 THE MANY FACES AND FORMS OF HORMONE REPLACEMENT THERAPY

ESTROGEN

Q: Estrogen and progestin seem to come in many shapes and sizes. Can you describe what's on the market and what's coming?

A: Certainly. Let's start with estrogen, which is available in pill, skin patch, cream and other forms. According to an ob-gyn at Vanderbilt University Medical Center, estrogen can also be combined with ordinary hand and body lotion.

The most popular form of estrogen is pill or tablet. When swallowed, oral estrogen is absorbed by the stomach and intestines, which send the estrogen via the bloodstream to the liver, where it is converted into estrone and then distributed to the tissues in the body.

Q: Sounds like oral estrogen is easy to use. Is that true?

A: Yes. However, women with stomach or intestinal disorders may not be able to absorb enough to make HRT effective. And because oral estrogen stimulates the liver, estrogen pills may be unsuitable for women with liver disease, high blood pressure, gallbladder disease or blood-clotting disorders. These women may choose to use a newer form of estrogen, the skin patch, or one of the other estrogen products.

Q: Can you tell me about the estrogen skin patch?

A: Sold as Estraderm, FemPatch, Climara and Vivelle, **transdermal estrogen** is applied much like a bandage to a clean, dry, nonoily, hairless area of the skin—preferably on the stomach, back, hip, thigh or buttock. The skin patch slowly releases estrogen, which is absorbed directly into the bloodstream without first passing through the liver.

Because the liver is bypassed, there is no apparent change in clotting factors (naturally occurring chemicals that affect the formation of blood clots) or in liver proteins, according to the *Physicians' Desk Reference.* For this reason, the patch is thought to be a better choice for women who can't take oral estrogen because it may aggravate medical conditions such as liver disease, high blood pressure, gallbladder disease and **thrombophlebitis** (a blood clot and inflammation in a vein in the leg). The patch can also be used by women who simply prefer applying a patch to taking a daily pill.

Q: Are there disadvantages to the patch?

A: Wearing the patch every day can irritate the skin. Adhesion may be a problem during hot, humid weather, and you must reapply or replace the patch if it falls off.

Q: How does vaginal estrogen cream work?

A: Vaginal estrogen cream is inserted into the vagina by means of an applicator that dispenses a measured amount of cream. With this form of estrogen, you follow a schedule devised by your doctor.

Like transdermal estrogen, vaginally applied estrogen is not absorbed through the digestive system and so does not pass through the liver, meaning that it is less likely to aggravate medical conditions such as liver disease, high blood pressure, gallbladder disease and thrombophlebitis.

Although *some* of the estrogen in the cream is absorbed into the bloodstream, most of it remains in the area of the vagina and urinary tract, helping to keep the tissues of the vagina and bladder firm and resilient and combating vaginal dryness and urinary tract infections in the years after menopause.

Vaginal suppositories made from finely ground estrogen are placed in the vagina and can be used instead of vaginal estrogen cream. They serve the same functions mentioned above.

Q: Can estrogen be taken by injection?

A: Yes. In the past, women who couldn't take estrogen orally might have been given intramuscular estrogen injections. Injections are rarely used today, made archaic by the advent of the transdermal patch.

Q: Are there any other forms of estrogen available?

A: There are several newer ways of delivering estrogen: **implanted subcutaneous estrogen pellets**, **buccal estrogen**, Estragel and **vaginal ring implants**. However, with the exception of vaginal ring implants, these methods are not currently approved for use in the United States.

Q: What are implanted subcutaneous estrogen pellets?

A: Estrogen pellets deliver estrogen to the bloodstream while bypassing the liver. Used in Europe, the pellets (or capsules) are surgically implanted just under the skin. They slowly release estrogen for six to 12 months. If you want to go off the hormone, however, the implant must be surgically removed. This estrogen delivery system is undergoing further research.

Q: What is buccal estrogen?

A: Buccal estrogen is a low-dose estrogen tablet that you place inside your mouth, against your cheek. As it dissolves, the estrogen is absorbed through the mucous membranes into the bloodstream. Although buccal estrogen is currently in use in Europe, final approval by the Food and Drug Administration (FDA) for use in the United States is pending.

Q: What is Estragel?

A: In France, women use an estrogen gel that is measured with an applicator and then rubbed on the abdomen. This estrogen is absorbed through the skin into the bloodstream. In the United States, research is ongoing into the use of estrogen gel for the treatment of moderate to severe vasomotor symptoms associated with menopause.

Q: You mentioned a vaginal ring implant. What is that?

A: A vaginal ring implant (brand name Estring) is inserted into the vagina by the woman and left there to slowly release set amounts of estrogen every 24 hours. This system delivers estrogen to the urogenital tissue as well as or better than estrogen cream, according to *Drug Topics.*

PROGESTERONE

Q: **Now I know the many forms of estrogen that are currently available or that may be available after approval. But what about progesterone? Didn't you say in earlier chapters that progesterone plays a role in hormone replacement therapy?**

A: Yes—a very important role. Regardless of the form it comes in, estrogen can encourage the buildup of endometrial tissue, sometimes leading to hyperplasia (a proliferation of cells in the endometrium that can set the stage for cancer). If you have a uterus, you'll probably need to take progestin—a synthetic or natural form of progesterone—to prevent this potentially dangerous condition. And there are a number of ways to do this: pill, suppository, gel or intrauterine device (IUD).

Q: **Can you tell me about oral progestin?**

A: Hormone replacement therapy (HRT), as practiced today, usually entails supplementing estrogen with oral progestin (progestin in pill form). The most commonly prescribed progestin is medroxyprogesterone acetate. Brand names include Amen, Cycrin and Provera.

Q: Didn't I read about a natural progesterone soon to be on the market?

A: You're talking about Prometrium, which is derived from wild yams and is chemically the same as the progesterone found in a woman's ovaries. This natural, micronized (finely ground) progesterone is reported to cause fewer of the troublesome side effects (see page 60)—which include symptoms common to premenstrual syndrome—associated with the progestins on the market today. Prometrium, the first natural progesterone pill, is awaiting FDA approval.

Q: Why do some women use progestin suppositories?

A: Progestin suppositories are available for women who are unable to take oral progestin. For instance, some women have stomach or intestinal disorders that prevent them from absorbing enough of the oral medication.

A progesterone gel (brand name Crinone) is also available as an "off label" medication for HRT. A single-use disposable unit containing a measured amount of finely ground progesterone is inserted vaginally once a day, every other day. This dose is absorbed and distributed to the uterus.

Q: You mentioned an intrauterine device. Can you tell me about it?

A: Progestasert is an intrauterine device that provides a very low, steady dose of progestin and eliminates the need for oral progestin. This is beneficial for women who need a localized form of progestin. According to Susan M. Love, M.D., in *Dr. Susan Love's Hormone Book,* "Like the lower doses of the vaginal creams, there's not enough to be absorbed into the body as a whole. This is based on the very sensible idea that where you really want the progesterone is in the uterus, so it can protect the endometrium."

APPROACHES AND FORMULATIONS

Q: Tell me again—what are the two approaches to HRT?

A: Current HRT involves taking estrogen alone (unopposed estrogen) or taking estrogen in combination with progestin (combination therapy).

As we said before, unopposed estrogen is estrogen given without any other hormone. (Generally, unopposed estrogen is prescribed only for women without a uterus.) Depending upon the regimen your doctor recommends, you may take estrogen for 21 days a month, 25 days a month or without interruption.

Q: Are there different pill formulations of unopposed estrogen?

A: Yes. The four commonly prescribed forms are **conjugated equine estrogen**, **esterified estrogen**, **micronized estradiol** and **estropipate**.

Q: What is conjugated equine estrogen?

A: The most popular pill formulation of estrogen, conjugated equine estrogen (sold as Premarin or in generic form) is derived from the urine of pregnant mares. In addition to its oral formulation, it's available as a vaginal cream and as an injection. The average oral dose of Premarin varies, depending upon its intended purpose. For treating hot flashes, for example, the dose is 0.3 to 1.25 milligrams (mg.) daily for 20 consecutive days each month. For treating osteoporosis, the dose is 0.625 mg. daily in cycles (three weeks on, one week off). The average vaginal dose is 2 to 4 grams (g.) daily in cycles (three weeks on, one week off).

Q: What should I know about the other common pill formulations of estrogen?

A: Esterified estrogen (Estratab and Menest) is a natural form of estrogen. The average dose is 0.3 to 1.25 mg. or more daily in cycles (three weeks on, one week off).

Micronized estradiol (Estrace) is a finely ground form of estrogen. In addition to pill form, it's also available as a transdermal (skin) patch and as a vaginal cream.

Q: Wait a minute—what's the typical dosage and regimen?

A: The dose will be different for different women. And even after a woman's doctor has determined the correct dosage, modifications may be necessary as the woman's body adjusts to the dosage. Having said that, the average dose of Estrace in pill form is 1 to 2 mg. daily in cycles (21 days on, seven days off *or* five days on, two days off).

The average dose of Estrace as a skin patch is one patch delivering 0.05 mg. every 24 hours, applied twice a week in cycles (three weeks on, one week off).

The average dose of Estrace as a vaginal cream is 2 to 4 g. daily for one to two weeks, then 1 g. one to three times a week in cycles.

Q: OK. Now what about estropipate?

A: Estropipate is a synthetic form of estrogen (sold in pill form as Ogen and Ortho-Est). The average oral dose of estropipate is 0.625 mg. daily. The average vaginal dose is 2 to 4 g. daily in cycles (three weeks on, one week off).

COMBINATION HRT

Q: **Let's move on to combination HRT. So progestin is added to one of the forms of estrogen we just talked about, right?**

A: Right—and for one simple reason: Progestin protects the uterus. You see, constant estrogen stimulation causes the lining of the uterus, the endometrium, to grow and thicken.

Q: **If the endometrium gets too thick, hyperplasia can result, and that sometimes develops into endometrial cancer. Is that what you've been saying?**

A: That's correct. Progestin works to prevent the uterine lining from reaching dangerously thick levels, thus forestalling the risk of endometrial cancer. For this reason, most women with uteruses are advised to take progestin along with estrogen. Women who have had hysterectomies don't need progestin.

Q: **Can you explain the dosages and different regimens for combination HRT?**

A: Yes. There are four common estrogen-progestin combination regimens: **cyclic sequential therapy**, **cyclic combined therapy**, **continuous sequential therapy** and **continuous combined therapy**.

Q: Let's start with cyclic sequential therapy.
What is it?

A: In cyclic sequential therapy, 0.625 mg. of conjugated
estrogen (or an equivalent) is taken for 21 or 25 days
of the month, with 5 to 10 mg. of progestin added to the estrogen daily for the last 10 to 14 days. Then nothing is taken for
five days. Cyclic sequential therapy is designed to mimic the
menstrual cycle. During the first few years of using estrogen
and cyclic progestin, a woman experiences two to three days
of monthly bleeding followed by light spotting, much like a
normal menstrual period.

Q: What is cyclic combined therapy?

A: The woman takes 0.625 mg. of conjugated estrogen
(or an equivalent) and a low dose (2.5 mg.) of progestin for 25 days each month, with a five- to six-day rest
period. This is a somewhat newer form of combination therapy,
and preliminary studies of its effectiveness show that there is
less unexpected light spotting or bleeding, called breakthrough
bleeding, compared with continuous combined therapy. (Breakthrough bleeding and related side effects of HRT are discussed
later in this chapter.)

Q: Before we get to continuous combined therapy,
you had also mentioned continuous sequential
therapy. What is that?

A: A woman takes 0.625 mg. of conjugated estrogen
(or an equivalent) every day of the month. Progestin
(10 mg. of medroxyprogesterone or 2.5 to 5 mg. of norethindrone or norethindrone acetate) is taken for 12 to 14 days,
from the 12th through the 25th day of the month. As with
cyclic sequential therapy, there is menstrual-like bleeding at
the end of the month.

Q: OK. Now, what is continuous combined therapy?

A: In this treatment, 0.625 mg. of estrogen (or an equivalent) and varying amounts of progestin (2.5 mg., 5 mg. or 10 mg.)—depending upon the practitioner's advice—are taken every day of the month. The form of progestin generally used is medroxyprogesterone acetate.

This therapy is designed to prevent the menstrual-like bleeding (which many women dislike) of cyclic sequential and continuous sequential therapies. The trade-off, however, is that many women (40 percent after six months) continue to experience up to 20 days of light breakthrough bleeding each month.

Q: So does a woman have to take two pills every day with combination therapy?

A: Actually, no. Prempro is a popular continuous combined therapy in one tablet.

Q: How much estrogen and progestin does Prempro have in it?

A: A pill with 0.625 mg. of conjugated estrogen and 2.5 mg. of medroxyprogesterone is available. In addition, a newer, stronger formulation—Prempro with 0.625 mg. of conjugated estrogen and 5 mg. of medroxyprogesterone—was recently approved for women who need more progestin to achieve amenorrhea (cessation of menstrual-like bleeding associated with HRT).

Q: Are there any other types of combination therapy I should know about?

A: One other—estrogen plus testosterone, which includes a small dose of testosterone, an **androgen** (a steroid

hormone that increases growth of male physical characteristics). It is sometimes prescribed to women who have had their
ovaries and uteruses surgically removed, as well as to women
in perimenopause—the early stages of menopause—who
report a loss of sexual desire.

Testosterone increases sexual desire. It can also help relieve
breast tenderness, one of the short-term side effects of estrogen
therapy, according to Ronald L. Young, M.D., of Baylor College
of Medicine in Houston.

Estratest, an esterified estrogen (1.25 mg. daily) with methyltestosterone (1.25 or 2.5 mg. daily), and a version of Premarin
(0.625 mg. conjugated estrogen daily) with methyltestosterone
(1.25 mg. daily) are two such drugs on the market. If it turns
out that you are a candidate for estrogen-testosterone therapy,
be sure to talk with your practitioner about the side effects
unique to testosterone—namely, cosmetic and lipid (blood
fat) side effects.

HOW MUCH TO TAKE
AND FOR HOW LONG

Q: If I decide to go on HRT, how much estrogen
should I take?

A: Good question. But before we answer and discuss
several factors influencing what is the right dose for
you, let us say this: The general medical philosophy is that you
should take the lowest dose that works. The more estrogen
and progestin you take, the greater your risk of developing
uncomfortable and potentially dangerous side effects. According to the May 1998 American College of Obstetricians and
Gynecologists (ACOG) Educational Bulletin, "The lowest effective estrogen dose that will relieve the patient's symptoms and
provide cardiovascular and bone protection should be used."
Your doctor may recommend the standard 0.625 mg. dose or
a lower dose that suits your needs.

Some women get relief from menopausal symptoms with only 0.3 mg. of estrogen a day. In 1998, the FDA approved a 0.3 mg. version of Estratab, a plant-derived estrogen, to help protect against osteoporosis with fewer side effects. According to the FDA and the drug's manufacturer, low-dose Estratab doesn't appear to affect the uterus in the same way that higher-dose estrogen does.

Q: **What determines how much estrogen is right for me?**

A: Six factors can help determine this.

- *How much estrogen your body produced during your reproductive years.* The only way to know these numbers, however, is to have your blood tested for estradiol levels before you enter the menopausal years. If you're already experiencing menopause, it's too late to get these measurements.

- *Your age.* Younger women may need twice as much estrogen as older women to alleviate symptoms, according to the *Cecil Textbook of Medicine.*

- *Your weight.* Heavier women may need smaller doses because they have more estrone—the estrogen produced from fat cells—in their bodies than thinner women.

- *Whether your menopause was surgical or natural.* Women who have had their ovaries surgically removed may need higher estrogen amounts. Because of the suddenness of surgical menopause, these women tend to have more severe menopausal symptoms than women who have had natural menopause.

- *Whether you smoke.* Smoking has been found to reduce the amounts of estradiol and estrone in the blood. So cigarette smokers on HRT appear to need higher doses of estrogen, according to research published in *Obstetrics and Gynecology.*

- *Your body's sensitivity to estrogen in general.* You can determine this only by trying the standard dose of estrogen and seeing how you react. If you're still experiencing side effects such as headaches, breast pain or swelling after four months, you may need a lower dose or a different estrogen formulation. Each pharmaceutical estrogen—conjugated, esterified, micronized—has a different formulation and affects individual women a little differently. If you take HRT and it doesn't relieve your symptoms, your doctor may increase the dosage for several months. Finding the right dose of estrogen (and the right ratio of estrogen to progestin, if you take combined therapy) that works for you is part science and part guesswork.

Q: **So much for estrogen. But what about progestin? How much should I take?**

A: It depends, as we've already shown (see pages 104-105). If, for example, you are on cyclic sequential therapy, the rule of thumb is 5 to 10 mg. of a progestin such as medroxyprogesterone acetate, taken for 10 to 14 consecutive days of the month. If you are on, say, continuous combined therapy, you may be prescribed 2.5 mg., 5 mg. or 10 mg. daily throughout the month. The 10 mg. dose is thought to provide the best protection against developing hyperplasia and endometrial cancer, but it also causes more side effects, such as headaches and depression. Reaching the right balance of estrogen and progestin may require some dose adjustments in the first few months of treatment.

Q: **If I decide to take long-term preventive hormone therapy, when should I begin?**

A: We talked about this a little in chapter 3. If you decide to take preventive HRT, your doctor may suggest beginning estrogen replacement within three years of your last men-strual period—and may recommend continuing it for life, if you are extremely concerned about or at high risk of osteoporosis or heart disease. If you want to protect yourself against either or both of these conditions but are concerned about the risks of long-term HRT (which we discuss in the following chapter), your practitioner may suggest seven to 10 years of therapy. But remember—not all experts agree on what's best.

"There are going to be benefits whenever you start," says Rogerio A. Lobo, M.D., in *Scientific American Presents: Women's Health* (Summer 1998). Graham A. Colditz, M.D., an outspoken critic of estrogen therapy, counters, "[The issue of when to start] is really a central question that still hasn't been answered. If you start at age 65 rather than at age 50, is the benefit still there? Because after all, the risk of heart attack and hip fracture between ages 50 and 60 is in fact pretty small. Because few women have started taking hormones at older ages, there's not a lot of experience yet. [The bone benefits] may not be as pronounced as they would be for someone who began taking hormones earlier in life, but there should still be benefits."

Q: OK. Let's say I decide to take HRT long-term as a preventive. Which form should I take?

A: HRT—either estrogen alone or in combination with progestin—offers protection against heart disease. If you understand the risks of taking estrogen alone, you can elect to use it—provided you commit to physical exams once or twice a year and an annual endometrial biopsy to test your endometrium's health.

If you choose combination therapy, you can select estrogen and progestin in the cyclic therapy or estrogen and progestin in the continuous therapy. Current evidence suggests that the cyclic therapy offers better protection for the heart, while the continuous therapy is preferred by many women because it does not cause monthly menstrual-like bleeding.

Q: Is there a specific form of estrogen I should use for long-term preventive hormone therapy?

A: Depending upon what you hope to achieve with long-term hormone therapy, you have the full range of HRT products to choose from. Most of the current research has focused on oral estrogen, so comparatively less is known about the effectiveness of patches, creams, injections and other, newer forms of estrogen distribution. Research suggests that estrogen in pill form may give a better boost to HDL (high-density lipoprotein), the "good" cholesterol, than the trans-dermal patch. However, if you can't take oral estrogen because of health considerations, then you may have to use the patch and know that it may be less effective in certain cases.

SHORT-TERM SIDE EFFECTS

Q: Judging from what HRT can do to help alleviate menopausal symptoms and the precise regimens involved in it, I assume that hormones are powerful drugs. Can we talk about side effects now?

A: Certainly. Some of the possible short-term side effects associated with combination therapy include **withdrawal bleeding**, breakthrough bleeding, water retention and bloating, breast swelling and tenderness, nausea and/or abdominal cramps, weight gain, chronic headaches, and depression and irritability.

Women taking unopposed estrogen experience similar, though less extensive, side effects. And we already mentioned that the skin patch may cause a rash, irritation and redness at the patch site.

Q: You mentioned menstrual-like bleeding here and earlier. Doesn't that stop when a woman is menopausal?

A: If you're taking combination therapy in a cyclic or sequential regimen—that is, estrogen with progestin on certain days of the month—then your most prominent side effect will be the return of your menstrual periods. Doctors call this withdrawal bleeding because it occurs after progestin is discontinued, or withdrawn, each month. Eighty to 90 percent of women who begin taking cyclic estrogen plus progestin resume their periods, which most women aren't too keen about. Bleeding is listed as the primary reason why women decide not to begin HRT, as well as a major reason why they discontinue it.

Q: What is the bleeding like?

A: The bleeding mimics the menstrual periods you had when you were younger. Each month, withdrawal bleeding removes the buildup of blood and endometrial tissue caused by taking estrogen, thus cleaning your uterus. These periods generally last from two to five days and gradually lighten over time. After six months to a year of HRT, for example, you may experience only a couple of days of spotting. Eventually, the periods disappear.

Q: Does regaining my period mean I can get pregnant?

A: No. HRT won't reactivate your ovaries once they have stopped releasing eggs.

Q: **Will I also have withdrawal bleeding if I take continuous combined therapy?**

A: You may have light menstrual-like spotting (breakthrough bleeding) during the first six months of treatment. But because you take progestin continually, you won't experience the withdrawal bleeding that women on the cyclic combined regimen have.

Q: **What if the breakthrough bleeding lasts for more than a few days?**

A: Report any breakthrough bleeding to your practitioner, who may decide to adjust the ratio of estrogen to progestin. If the bleeding lasts for more than 10 days or is heavier than your normal menstrual periods ever were, your doctor may perform tests such as an endometrial biopsy or an ultrasound to rule out cervical polyps (small, usually noncancerous growths), uterine **fibroids** (noncancerous muscle and tissue growths) or hyperplasia.

Q: **You listed some other short-term side effects. Can you explain them?**

A: Sure. Here's a look at some side effects.

- *Water retention and bloating.* Half of the women who take HRT experience fluid retention or feelings of gas and bloatedness, caused by both estrogen and progestin. If these side effects don't pass in a few weeks and you find them bothersome, speak to your doctor. She may adjust your hormone dose, suggest altering your intake of salt and caffeine (which encourage water retention), offer a prescription diuretic (a drug that promotes the production and discharge of urine) or recommend taking a small amount of a natural diuretic such as vitamin B_6.

- *Breast swelling and tenderness.* Women who take HRT often develop swollen and tender breasts, similar to premenstrual breast tenderness. Called **mastalgia**, it is thought to be triggered by estrogen. It may disappear in a few months. Your doctor might choose to lower your estrogen dose or prescribe a combination of estrogen and testosterone to relieve painful breasts.

- *Nausea and/or abdominal cramps.* Some women who take combination HRT have nausea or cramping in the lower abdomen during and after the days they take progestin. Taking smaller doses of progestin may eliminate this.

- *Weight gain.* At least 25 percent of women who use HRT put on weight, particularly in the breasts, lower abdomen and hips, according to some experts. Some of the gain may be caused by the fluid retained during the first few months of using HRT. (Other causes of weight gain are not necessarily attributable to HRT, including a slowdown in the body's metabolism that accompanies aging and a reduction in calorie burning due to a lower level of exercise.) Some doctors believe that estrogen itself tends to encourage the development of fat tissue; others do not agree. Adjusting dosage may or may not help.

Q: A friend of mine says her headaches were caused by HRT. Is this possible?

A: Some women on HRT report that they develop chronic headaches. Researchers think that the cause is fluid retention in the brain. Usually, headaches disappear after three to four months of therapy. If they continue, however, your doctor may need to reduce the amount of estrogen you're taking.

If you're prone to migraines, the estrogen in HRT may increase the number you experience. If so, you may need to stop taking estrogen altogether. (We have more to say about migraines and HRT in chapter 5.)

Q: Are there any more side effects I should know about?

A: If you find yourself feeling depressed or irritated after beginning HRT, your doctor may reduce your progestin dose, have you try a different form of progestin or give you a prescription for natural progesterone (which, at least for now, must be prepared by a pharmacist). Natural progesterone is thought to be less likely to provoke depression than synthetic progestin. In fact, trying different forms of estrogen and progestin may be useful in addressing all HRT side effects.

Other reported reactions to HRT include rashes, increased appetite, increased vaginal secretions, lower levels of sexual desire—and, conversely, heightened sexual desire. Clearly, there's a great and even conflicting range of side effects.

Q: Is there any relief from these side effects?

A: Some reactions are eliminated by adjusting (usually reducing) the dosage of estrogen and/or progestin. Other reactions disappear after six to eight months of hormone use, as your body adjusts to the new types of drugs in its system. Still other side effects can be managed through diet and exercise or by taking additional medications. All of them disappear if you stop using HRT.

Q: What about long-terms effects of HRT?

A: We discuss long-term effects of HRT in chapter 5, along with **absolute contraindications** and **relative contraindications**—situations and medical conditions that prohibit the use of HRT and situations and medical conditions under which HRT should be used with great care and medical supervision.

5 THE RISKS OF LONG-TERM HORMONE REPLACEMENT THERAPY

Q: What are the risks of long-term hormone replacement therapy?

A: No clear evidence currently exists about how long-term hormone replacement therapy (HRT) affects the body. As mentioned in chapter 4, short-term side effects of estrogen and progestin can include withdrawal and breakthrough bleeding, water retention and bloating, breast swelling and tenderness, nausea and lower abdominal cramps, weight gain, chronic headaches and others. Long-term side effects, however, are less clear. Possible ones include endometrial cancer, breast cancer, **thromboembolic disease** and liver and gallbladder problems.

Q: Why are long-term side effects less clear?

A: Although HRT has been around in some form for 60 or so years, the long-term hazards of taking HRT are matters of intense medical debate due to the lack of consensus among the many studies. At least one hazard, endometrial cancer, has been linked to unopposed estrogen. But information on the impact of combination therapy, the most popular form of HRT today, is just coming to light. Some of this information will not be released until the next century.

ENDOMETRIAL CANCER

Q: Can you tell me a little about endometrial cancer?

A: According to 1998 figures from the National Cancer Institute, approximately 36,100 new cases of endometrial (uterine) cancer develop each year, and about 6,300 women die from endometrial cancer annually. It is the fourth most common form of cancer in women.

Q: Who is at greatest risk of developing endometrial cancer?

A: At greatest risk is a woman with a uterus who takes unopposed estrogen for 10 or more years. She has a four- to 10-fold greater risk of developing endometrial cancer than a woman who doesn't take the hormone. That increased risk persists for five to 15 years after HRT is stopped, according to Elizabeth Barrett-Connor, M.D., writing in the *Annual Review of Medicine.* However, says Barrett-Connor, endometrial cancer usually is caught early and generally has an excellent survival rate. But you wouldn't want to be the exception— nor would you want to develop cancer at all.

Q: How does estrogen cause cancer?

A: Estrogen itself does not cause cancer. As you may recall, estrogen promotes the potentially dangerous precancerous condition called hyperplasia.

Q: Does all hyperplasia develop into cancer?

A: No. Hyperplasia can develop into cancer if it is neglected and if you are predisposed to uterine cancer. A family history of endometrial cancer is a warning flag, as is obesity. Women who are more than 20 percent overweight have a slightly greater risk of endometrial cancer.

Q: Why are these overweight women at greater risk?

A: Fat cells produce estrone, a form of estrogen. Overweight women have an abundance of fat cells, which means these women have greater amounts of estrogen in their bodies than women at or below their proper weights.

Q: Are there other risk factors?

A: Yes. Other risk factors may include conditions such as diabetes, high cholesterol and high blood pressure. But the greatest risk factor appears to be taking unopposed estrogen. The Postmenopausal Estrogen/Progestin Interventions Trial examined the effects of estrogen taken alone. Over a three-year period, women who took 0.625 milligrams (mg.) of conjugated equine estrogen (derived from the urine of mares) were more likely to develop hyperplasia than women who took a placebo, or inactive substance. Women who took estrogen in combination with progesterone had the same rate of hyperplasia as women who took a placebo.

Q: If I take a lower dose of estrogen, will that decrease my risk of endometrial cancer?

A: Not necessarily. Although most doctors prescribe the lowest amount of unopposed estrogen possible, researchers are unsure whether this makes much of a difference. According to a recent study published in *Obstetrics and Gynecology,* women who took 0.3 mg. of unopposed estrogen daily for eight or more years had about the same risk of endometrial cancer as women who took the larger dose of 0.625 mg.

Q: What are the symptoms of hyperplasia?

A: The primary symptoms are unexpected (breakthrough) bleeding and unusually heavy or long-lasting bleeding. Be aware that hyperplasia can develop in the years before menopause, when your body's menstrual cycle becomes irregular and unpredictable. During the perimenopausal years, hyperplasia causes very heavy menstrual periods and/or breakthrough bleeding.

Q: Can a Pap test detect hyperplasia?

A: Not always. A Pap test checks the condition of the cervix, not the condition of the endometrium. Tests such as an endometrial biopsy or a **dilatation and curettage (D&C)**—a procedure in which the uterus is scraped clean—can determine if you have hyperplasia.

Q: Is there anything I can do to protect myself against endometrial cancer?

A: To fight the dangers of unopposed estrogen, doctors prescribe progestin in tandem with estrogen for women with uteruses. According to the May 1998 American College of Obstetricians and Gynecologists (ACOG) Educational Bulletin on HRT, cyclic or continuous therapy (see chapter 4) is required in women with uteruses to protect the endometrium from hyperplasia during HRT. As you may recall, progestin suppresses hyperplasia by preventing the thick uterine buildup.

In rare cases, hyperplasia can develop even if a woman is taking progestin—possibly because the woman is supersensitive to the effects of estrogen. Larger progestin doses may be needed. In short, even women on combination therapy still need to pay attention to unusual bleeding.

Q: **How often do I need to take progestin to help guard against hyperplasia and cancer?**

A: Although no one knows the precise minimum number of days you need to take progestin to reduce the risk of endometrial cancer, studies suggest that most women are protected if they take at least 12 days of progestin each month.

Q: **How much progestin should I take?**

A: According to the ACOG, some research studies suggest that taking at least 10 mg. of progestin for 12 days increases this hormone's effectiveness. The ACOG recommends that women with uteruses use cyclic or continuous progestin therapy to protect against hyperplasia during hormone replacement.

Q: **Is it ever possible to take unopposed estrogen?**

A: As mentioned previously, unopposed estrogen is the treatment of choice if you have had a hysterectomy. However, if you have a uterus and take progestin and find that you cannot tolerate progestin's side effects, you can continue to take unopposed estrogen. But you must commit to annual tests (usually an endometrial biopsy) to monitor the health of your endometrium. If the endometrium is found to be thicker than 4 millimeters (mm.), your doctor may order additional procedures such as a transvaginal ultrasound or a D&C to check for hyperplasia.

Q: Is there a way to treat hyperplasia?

A: When it's caught early, hyperplasia is usually treated with a two- to three-month course of progestin. This causes the uterus to completely and cleanly shed the built-up layer of cells in the endometrium, bringing down the endo-metrium's thickness so that it's within a normal range.

BREAST CANCER

Q: What can you tell me about breast cancer?

A: Let's start with the statistics. One in nine women in the United States will develop breast cancer in her lifetime. In 1998, nearly 180,000 cases of breast cancer were diagnosed in the United States, and more than 40,000 women died from the disease. In fact, breast cancer is the leading cause of cancer death in women between the ages of 40 and 55. The incidence of breast cancer increases with age, rising sharply after age 40. Nearly 80 percent of all breast cancers occur in women over age 50.

Q: What is the link between estrogen and breast cancer?

A: First, let us say that breast cancer is much more common in women than in men. Estrogen is known to affect breast tissue, occasionally encouraging abnormal cell growth and benign cysts in the breasts (fibrocystic breast disease). Some forms of breast cancer are estrogen dependent, meaning they grow in the presence of estrogen. Also, extensive tests have shown that estrogen is associated with the development of breast tumors in animals.

Q: So where does HRT fit into this issue?

A: You know, of course, that HRT includes estrogen, whether alone or in combination with progestin. The major question, then, is whether HRT increases a woman's risk of breast cancer. Frankly, this is a matter of great controversy. On one side of the debate are those who say that the vast body of scientific research has found little or no connection between HRT and breast cancer. On the other side are those who point to studies suggesting that HRT may increase the risk of breast cancer in postmenopausal women.

And complicating the mix of fact and opinion is the idea that for many women, the benefits of HRT do not compensate for the fear of acquiring breast cancer.

Q: What have the studies found?

A: The Nurses' Health Study, a massive study of registered nurses begun in 1976 and continuing today, has found both benefits and risks in HRT use by postmenopausal women. Specifically in the area of breast cancer, the Nurses' Health Study indicates that long-term HRT use (10 years of treatment) increases the risk of dying from breast cancer by 43 percent.

A recent analysis of research on HRT and breast cancer, published in *Lancet,* also found a possible connection. Fifty-one studies involving more than 52,000 women with breast cancer and 108,000 women without the disease were evaluated. This so-called meta-analysis concluded that using HRT for five or more years increases the risk of breast cancer by 35 percent. However, the increased risk disappears five years after women stop taking the hormones.

Critics of this meta-analysis contend that it didn't include enough information on specific HRT preparations, whether estrogen alone or combination hormone therapy.

Yet according to the ACOG, "Although some studies have suggested that HRT is linked to an increased risk of breast cancer in postmenopausal women, other studies have shown little or no relationship between estrogen use and breast cancer.... No consistent link between hormone replacement therapy and breast cancer has been found."

And so the debate continues. Clearly, the question of whether the risks of HRT outweigh the benefits remains open to further research. Just remember, though, that the higher risks do not predict that most women on HRT will develop cancer.

Q: In terms of benefits, are you talking about the effects of HRT on a woman's risk of heart disease?

A: Yes, primarily. No doubt you are referring to our discussion in chapter 3 and to studies that have found that women taking HRT are at significantly decreased risk of developing heart disease.

Q: Back to breast cancer—aren't there other risk factors at play?

A: Many experts claim that estrogen in and of itself doesn't cause breast cancer; they claim that other risk factors must be present. These factors increase the relative risk of breast cancer, meaning that the risk applies to a statistical sampling of women and may or may not apply to you in particular. The risk factors include the following:

- Family history of breast cancer

- Early menstruation

- First childbirth after age 30

- Obesity

- Inactive lifestyle

- Smoking

- High-fat diet

- Age

Q: **Can a woman use HRT to relieve menopausal symptoms if she had breast cancer years ago?**

A: The general consensus is that HRT is inappropriate for someone who is currently being treated for cancer. Medical experts disagree, however, about what is appropriate if a woman has a personal history of cancer. You see, many doctors are uncomfortable recommending HRT when its safety and benefit for successfully treated breast cancer patients have not been extensively tested in controlled clinical studies. The sticking point is this: In light of the difficulty in ascertaining that no dormant cancer remains in a woman's body, how does one define the cured or successfully treated cancer survivor?

A woman's individual practitioner, though, will have a personal point of view. The doctor may argue against HRT for women who have had cancer; or may suggest it for a very brief period to relieve extremely severe menopausal symptoms; or may agree that it is useful, under careful medical supervision, for women who have had cancer but who are also at high risk of osteoporosis or heart disease.

If you have had breast cancer and are weighing HRT use, it would be wise to get at least one other opinion from a highly respected cancer specialist or cancer center.

Q: Is there a relationship between progestin and breast cancer?

A: That is even less clear. Most studies have shown no link between progestin and breast cancer, some studies have found that progestin may increase breast cancer risk, and still others have shown that progestin may even reduce that risk. At present, most researchers think that progestin, taken for five or fewer years, doesn't increase breast cancer risk.

Q: From what you've told me, I don't think I'm at risk of breast cancer. I'd like to try HRT for its possible benefits. Any advice?

A: In making the HRT decision, you and your practitioner will want to weigh the possible increased risk of breast cancer against the possible osteoporotic and cardiovascular benefits of therapy. One thing to keep in mind: More women suffer from heart disease than breast cancer.

But for women at risk of breast cancer, the potential benefits of HRT do not allay fears. Thus, more and more women and their practitioners are reexamining whether HRT should be used for life or restricted in duration.

Q: All this information seems very conflicting. Will we ever know for certain if HRT increases the risk of breast cancer?

A: Unfortunately, the studies that we've briefly reviewed show why women and their doctors must assess individual risk factors. For now, we have to wait a while longer for better evidence.

In the meantime, the ACOG encourages women on HRT to do monthly breast self-examinations and to have a mammography every one to two years after age 40 and annually after age 50.

Q: You mentioned other conditions linked to HRT. Can you refresh my memory and tell me what they are?

A: Yes. Other possible long-term effects of HRT include thromboembolic disease and liver and gallbladder problems.

THROMBOEMBOLIC DISEASE

Q: What is thromboembolic disease?

A: *Thromboembolic disease* refers to any condition in which the body is more likely to form blood clots. A blood clot is known in scientific lingo as a **thrombus** or an **embolus** (although *embolus* can also refer to an object or a bit of tissue or gas in a blood vessel). When a thrombus forms in a blood vessel, the condition is known as thrombosis. When an embolus blocks a blood vessel, it is called an **embolism**.

Q: Blood clots can cause strokes, right?

A: Right—and heart attacks, too. In fact, blood clots are a major cause of both stroke and heart attack. A blood clot in an artery supplying the brain triggers a stroke. A blood clot in an artery supplying the heart triggers a heart attack. A blood clot in a vein produces an inflammation of the vein known as thrombophlebitis, which is one of the causes of varicose veins. Thrombophlebitis can be dangerous. If a blood clot breaks away from the wall of the blood vessel and travels to the heart, it may cause a heart attack.

Q: Does HRT increase the risk of blood clots?

A: The general consensus today is that HRT poses a risk only for women who have clear histories of thrombo-embolic disease or who have recently had blood clots. With attentive medical care, women with thrombophlebitis could take HRT.

Q: Why is HRT a problem for women with thromboembolic disease?

A: The answer may lie in the way estrogen affects the liver. Estrogen encourages the liver to produce sub-stances called clotting factors, chemicals within the body that cause bleeding to stop at the site of a cut or another injury. At the same time, estrogen encourages the liver to suppress the production of some anticlotting factors, chemicals that keep your blood from thickening. This usually isn't a problem for most women on the low doses of estrogen—especially conjugated equine estrogen—used in HRT today. It can be a problem for women who take estrogen at high doses, such as in some birth control pills.

Q: OK. You've said before that it's the oral form of HRT that affects the liver. Even though you haven't said so directly, you're implying that oral HRT shouldn't be used by women with thromboembolic disease. If this is the case, can't women with thromboembolic disease use a different type of HRT delivery system?

A: Yes, they can. Because oral estrogens can slightly alter the blood's clotting factors through hepatic (pertaining to the liver) stimulation, many experts now recommend that HRT be delivered through the skin patch. Discuss this with your practitioner if you have or are at risk of thromboembolic disease.

Q: Speaking of that—what are the risk factors for thromboembolic disease?

A: A family history of blood clotting, smoking, obesity, an earlier episode of thrombosis or embolism and severe varicose veins are some of the risk factors.

LIVER AND GALLBLADDER PROBLEMS

Q: Since the liver has been coming up a lot in our discussion, can you tell me more what the liver does?

A: The liver, a large gland located in the upper right region of your abdominal cavity, has many important jobs: secreting thick-fluid bile (sometimes called gall), producing blood-clotting substances, regulating blood sugar levels and neutralizing poisonous substances. The liver works together with the gallbladder, a reservoir for bile located on the lower side of the liver. Bile produced in the liver passes to the gallbladder, where it's stored until it's needed by the small intestine to break down fatty foods.

Q: How does HRT affect the liver?

A: When estrogen is taken orally, it's processed by the liver before it slips into the bloodstream. An impaired or diseased liver may not properly convert estrogen. As a result, estrogen may become a toxin in the body. Doctors believe that the hormones in vaginal estrogen creams and skin patches are safe because they are not taken orally and thus bypass the liver.

Q: How does HRT affect the gallbladder?

A: Estrogen—particularly oral estrogen—increases the odds of developing gallbladder disease. Estrogen encourages increased amounts of cholesterol to collect in the bile manufactured by the liver. When the bile becomes super-saturated with cholesterol, gallstones form. These stones usually are painful and sometimes require surgery.

Q: If a woman has a history of gallbladder problems, should she steer clear of HRT?

A: Again, it's oral estrogen that she should avoid. Skin patches and vaginal creams are thought to be safer because estrogen is absorbed through the bloodstream, bypassing the liver and the gallbladder.

But know this: Clinical studies haven't yet determined whether patches reduce the incidence of gallstones. If you have a history of gallbladder disease or gallstones and you choose to use HRT, be sure your doctor monitors the effects of the therapy on your body. If you develop gallstones during your course of HRT, then reevaluate your treatment regimen and perhaps change your diet (for example, by reducing your cholesterol intake).

OTHER POSSIBLE EFFECTS

Q: Are there connections between HRT and other health conditions?

A: Possibly. As hormone use comes under closer scrutiny, researchers are discovering possible connections between HRT and other health conditions. Among these conditions are hypertension, **ovarian cancer**, eye problems and uterine fibroids.

Q: Can you tell me a little bit about hypertension?

A: Certainly. Hypertension, or high blood pressure, occurs when the blood exerts a higher than normal force against artery walls. Two measurements are associated with blood pressure: systolic pressure (the higher of the two measurements) and diastolic pressure (the lower of the two measurements).

Q: What is considered high blood pressure?

A: Readings above 140/90 mm Hg (millimeters of mercury) over a period of time.

Q: How is HRT linked to hypertension?

A: Oral contraceptives that contain high doses of estrogen are known to increase the risk of hypertension. So naturally, the medical profession has carefully watched HRT for similar effects. You see, estrogen encourages the kidneys to produce **angiotensin**, a chemical that causes blood vessels to narrow. In turn, blood pressure can rise, a situation that doctors call estrogen-associated hypertension.

Some doctors believe that HRT may provoke high blood pressure or may make an existing case of hypertension worse, but other health professionals disagree. The ACOG points out that in research on women taking HRT for more than three years, close monitoring found no significant changes in the women's blood pressure.

As a precaution, women should have their blood pressure checked shortly after they start HRT, then have it checked regularly while they're on HRT. An article published in *Drug Topics* a few years back suggests that women who experience high blood pressure from oral estrogen might not have this problem with the skin patch.

Q: Does HRT cause ovarian cancer?

A: The possibility of a link between HRT and ovarian cancer was raised by Barrett-Connor in the *Annual Review of Medicine*. She notes that some studies from Britain have revealed areas of concern. One study found a 2.5-fold increase in ovarian cancer risk, with the highest risk associated with high doses of all types of estrogen.

However, several studies published within the past two years have shown that the link between estrogen therapy and ovarian cancer is not as strong as previously thought.

Q: What is the link between HRT and eye problems?

A: Some women who use estrogen skin patches after a total hysterectomy experience eye problems such as blurred or fluctuating vision; dry, itchy, burning, watery eyes; pain in the eye; and a pulling sensation within the eye, according to Andrew Gurwood, O.D., and his colleagues from the Pennsylvania College of Optometry, writing in *Optometry and Vision Science*.

See your doctor or an eye specialist if you experience such eye problems while using HRT.

Q: What is the connection between HRT and uterine fibroids?

A: First, let us say that fibroids are benign (noncancerous) tumors found in or on the uterus. Twenty percent of all women have fibroids, as do half of all women over age 50. Fibroids usually shrink on their own after menopause, when estrogen levels fall, says Sadja Greenwood, M.D., author of *Menopause, Naturally: Preparing for the Second Half of Life.*

Because estrogen stimulates fibroid growth, some women with large fibroids choose not to take HRT. Other women with fibroids wait two to three years before starting HRT to give their fibroids time to wither and shrink. Still other women are willing to try low-dose HRT, particularly if their fibroids are small and not troublesome.

Q: Wait a minute—how big can fibroids get? Should I be concerned?

A: Fibroids are seldom troublesome, so you might have one or more and not even know it. Sometimes, though, fibroids cause heavy bleeding during the menstrual cycle, cause pelvic pain or put uncomfortable pressure on the bladder or bowel. If fibroids grow large enough (three and one-half inches or more in diameter) or cause pain, your doctor may recommend surgery to remove the fibroids or an estrogen-blocking drug to shrink them.

Q: What if I go on HRT and then develop fibroids?

A: If the fibroids cause heavy bleeding, abdominal pain or uncomfortable pressure on your bladder or bowel, then you'll have to discontinue HRT. You probably won't be able to resume estrogen use.

Q: Is HRT related to any other health problems?

A: Possibly. A small study of 34 women with epilepsy found that 16 of the women experienced a decrease in their seizures during menopause. None of these women was taking estrogen. But among eight women who were taking HRT, six reported a worsening of their seizures.

Researchers at the Comprehensive Epilepsy Center at Cornell Medical Center, where the study was done, believe that the decrease in estrogen production during menopause may lessen seizures in some epileptic women. HRT may, in turn, worsen seizures.

Q: Does this mean that women with epilepsy shouldn't use HRT?

A: Women with epilepsy shouldn't be scared off from using HRT. The researchers speculate that adding low-dose progesterone may modify the effects of estrogen and help women with epilepsy who are sensitive to HRT use it more safely.

ABSOLUTE AND RELATIVE CONTRAINDICATIONS

Q: Are there circumstances in which HRT shouldn't be taken?

A: Yes. HRT is inappropriate if you have certain medical conditions. In medical lingo, these conditions are known as absolute contraindications to HRT. But before we begin, let us say that the issue of contraindications is controversial.

Q: Why is that?

A: Because many studies on HRT conflict. Conditions that were once considered absolute contraindications may not be so today. At the very least, some of these conditions are now considered relative contraindications, or situations in which HRT use must be weighed carefully.

Added to this is the general lack of consensus among medical practitioners, who don't agree when HRT is contraindicated. The best advice we can offer is that you and your practitioner weigh the benefits and risks of HRT. With that said, let's explore absolute and relative contraindications.

Absolute Contraindications

Q: OK. Which medical conditions would qualify as absolute contraindications?

A: There are several conditions that should flash a red light to any woman considering HRT.

- *Known or suspected estrogen-dependent cancer.* Certain cancers are estrogen dependent. These include uterine, kidney and some forms of breast cancer. Because you may not know if you have uterine or breast cancer, your doctor may recommend screening tests (such as an endometrial biopsy and a mammogram) before you begin HRT.

- *History of thromboembolic disease.* According to the May 1998 American College of Obstetricians and Gynecologists (ACOG) Educational Bulletin, "Recent studies have shown a two- to fourfold increase in the risk of venous thromboembolism in users of estrogen-only and combined estrogen-progestin hormone replacement therapy." However, the ACOG admits that the absolute risk of blood clots in both women who use estrogen and women who don't is low. Other sources advise women with recent histories of blood clots not to use HRT.

- *Active liver disease or impaired liver function.* As we said before, oral estrogen is processed by the liver before it goes into the bloodstream. A diseased or impaired liver may not convert estrogen properly; in turn, the estrogen may become a toxin in the body. A past history of liver disease, however, is not necessarily an absolute contraindication. Some doctors believe that vaginal estrogen creams and skin patches are safe for women who do not have active liver disease because these systems of estrogen delivery bypass the liver.

- *Undiagnosed vaginal bleeding.* If you're bleeding and you don't know why, you shouldn't start HRT before your practitioner investigates and addresses the problem. Vaginal bleeding can be a sign of uterine fibroids, hyperplasia, uterine cancer or cervical cancer. As you already know, estrogen can worsen these conditions. Undiagnosed bleeding may be eliminated as a contraindication if your doctor identifies its cause and finds that it's not affected by hormone use.

Relative Contraindications

Q: Which conditions are considered relative contraindications?

A: There are several, some of which we've already discussed. If you have one of the following conditions and you elect to take hormones, proceed with care. Work with your doctor to weigh the severity of your menopausal symptoms and the therapy's potential benefits in light of the following known risks. And make sure your doctor closely monitors your use of hormones and is ready to change your regimen if necessary.

With that said, here are the relative contraindications and brief summaries of the consensus of opinion.

- *High blood pressure.* HRT may cause blood pressure to rise or make existing hypertension worse.

- *Gallbladder disease.* Oral estrogen has been linked to gallbladder disease. Thus, your practitioner may recommend a skin patch or vaginal cream as your form of HRT.

- *Fibroids.* You may not want to use HRT if you have large fibroids or experience heavy bleeding, abdominal pain or uncomfortable pressure on your bladder or bowel.

- *Migraines.* Estrogen replacement in menopause can provoke migraines. Reducing the amount of estrogen you take may solve the problem. But if your migraines persist for several weeks after trying a lowered dose, you may decide that the benefits of hormone use are not worth the pain.

- *Endometriosis.* **Endometriosis,** which can be very painful, occurs when cells from the endometrium (the tissue lining the uterus) move outside the uterus and grow on other organs within the abdomen when stimulated by the menstrual cycle. Before menopause, treatment for this condition involves taking doses of estrogen, progestin and sometimes other hormones. If these don't work, the uterus, fallopian tubes and ovaries may be surgically removed. After menopause, less severe endometriosis may disappear when estrogen and progesterone levels fall. For this reason, doctors often withhold HRT from women with endometriosis for three to 12 months after menopause.

Q: Are there other conditions considered to be relative contraindications?

A: Yes. These include seizure disorders, congestive heart failure, high blood triglycerides and a history of diethyl-stilbestrol (DES, a potent estrogen) use by you or your mother.

Q: What if I try HRT and later decide that I don't want to take it? Do I have to continue using it?

A: No, but discuss the situation with your practitioner.

DISCONTINUING THERAPY

Q: Wait a minute—are you saying that I can't just stop HRT?

A: That's correct. Discuss your concerns with your doctor, who can propose alternatives and recommend ways to gently wean you off HRT. Don't try to adjust your medication without your doctor's approval. That can be dangerous. For example, if you still have your uterus, it's risky to stop taking progestin and continue taking unopposed estrogen.

Q: I'm curious. What would happen if I suddenly stopped HRT?

A: An abrupt cutoff can put you into full-fledged estrogen withdrawal, complete with severe menopausal symptoms such as hot flashes—the very thing many women take HRT to avoid. These occur for the same reason that original menopausal symptoms occur—a sudden and sharp drop in estrogen levels.

Q: If I taper off HRT as my doctor advises, will I still have recurring menopausal symptoms?

A: Maybe. Some women experience hot flashes even if they gradually phase out HRT. These symptoms are usually temporary. So in the same manner in which you and your doctor had to fine-tune your estrogen-progestin doses when you started HRT, some adjusting of hormones may be needed as you taper off.

Q: How exactly do I taper off?

A: Your practitioner may suggest slowing the frequency of taking estrogen, recommending that you take it every second or third day. Or she may prescribe a smaller dose or ask you to halve or quarter the estrogen pill. A patch can be cut into smaller pieces and applied as usual. It may take your body three to four months to adjust to the declining estrogen levels.

Q: Will I also have to cut back on progestin?

A: No. If you have been taking progestin, you'll probably be told to continue at the usual dose until you are finished with the estrogen. As long as you are taking estrogen, you'll need to guard against hyperplasia.

Q: If I change my mind, can I go back to using HRT?

A: In most cases, yes. You can almost always restart hormone therapy at a later date, under the guidance of your practitioner.

PRACTITIONERS WHO PROVIDE HRT

Q: You've alluded a lot to the importance of working with my practitioner. But I'm wondering— what type of doctor should I see to discuss HRT?

A: Clearly, you should see a practitioner who is very knowledgeable in the area of HRT. HRT regimens are very complex. Not only does the practitioner have to select the appropriate form of HRT—pill, patch or cream—for your needs, but she also has to determine the correct dose, monitor any risk factors that you may have and ensure that you are receiving the necessary nutrients (such as calcium) to make HRT effective. In addition, estrogen and progestin doses may change over time.

Q: What are my choices in practitioners?

A: Here are some of your choices.

- *Obstetrician/gynecologist (ob-gyn).* This is an M.D. (doctor of medicine) or a D.O. (doctor of osteopathy) trained in all aspects of pregnancy and childbirth, as well as in the health and proper functioning of the female reproductive system. Ob-gyns, by the way, are more likely to prescribe HRT than any other medical practitioners.

- *Family practitioner.* This is an M.D. or a D.O. trained in total health care of the individual (woman or man, adult or child) and the family. If you choose a family practitioner to oversee your HRT, be sure the doctor has knowledge and expertise in gynecology and in the health concerns of older women.

- *Internist.* This M.D. or D.O. specializes in the diagnosis and nonsurgical treatment of disease, especially disease in adults. Many internists set up practices in which they act as highly trained family doctors.

- *Endocrinologist.* This doctor is an M.D. or a D.O. specially trained in the treatment of hormonal disorders, including not only problems related to menopause but also diabetes, pituitary diseases and sexual problems. The usual track is for the physician to specialize in internal medicine with a subspecialty in endocrinology.

Q: Aren't there nurses or nurse specialists who can provide such care?

A: Yes. A *certified nurse-midwife* is a registered nurse who has completed graduate training in women's health, obstetrical care and gynecological care and who has passed an extensive credentialing examination administered by the American College of Nurse-Midwives. All 50 states allow certified nurse-midwives to practice, and in the vast majority of states, certified nurse-midwives have the authority to prescribe oral contraceptives and HRT.

Also, as a registered nurse with additional graduate training, a *nurse-practitioner* can give you information about HRT's pros and cons and about health-promoting steps for your postmenopausal years. Licensing laws vary from state to state, but in general, you can find a nurse-practitioner in an ob-gyn office or at a women's health center.

Q: OK. If I decide against HRT, can I try anything else?

A: Yes. If you decide that HRT is not for you and that you want to try something besides or in addition to diet and nutrition, exercise and medication to treat menopausal symptoms and *possibly* prevent osteoporosis and heart disease, you may want to consider the alternative therapies that we discuss in the next chapter.

6 ALTERNATIVE THERAPIES TO HORMONE REPLACEMENT THERAPY

Q: What are alternative therapies?

A: First, let us say that the combination of diet, vitamin and mineral supplementation, and exercise can be seen as an alternative or adjunct to hormone replacement therapy (HRT). With that said, alternative therapies, also known as complementary therapies, encompass a wide range of healing philosophies and practices usually considered to be outside the scope of mainstream medicine. Alternative therapies include treatments and approaches that are not typically taught in traditional medical schools or used in hospitals.

Generally speaking, alternative therapies view all parts of a person—physical, mental, emotional and spiritual—as harmoniously interrelated. Any disharmony is thought to burden the body and possibly lead to sickness.

Q: Which forms of alternative therapy can help women during menopause?

A: Many alternative therapies are available to help women take care of their health before, during and after the menopausal years. They include, but are not limited to, **homeopathy**, **naturopathy**, **herbal medicine**, **acupuncture** and **acupressure**, and **biofeedback**.

Keep in mind that few alternative therapies have been tested in clinical studies. Many people assume that all natural remedies and herbal medicines, the main tools of alternative therapies, are safe. According to Wulf H. Utian, M.D., author of *Managing Your Menopause,* the proper dosages of some natural products are not known because they have not been tested like prescription and nonprescription drugs.

HOMEOPATHY

Q: What can you tell me about homeopathy?

A: Homeopathy, or **homeopathic medicine**, developed in the late eighteenth century. It's a system of medicine founded on the idea that the whole person must be treated, not just the condition. Therefore, symptoms indicate that a woman's life force is imbalanced, and that balance must be restored for a healthy body, mind and spirit.

Homeopathy treats illness by using very tiny, safe doses of medicines extracted from natural sources—such as plants, animal materials and natural chemicals—that stimulate a woman's own healing powers while avoiding harmful side effects.

Q: How can homeopathy treat menopausal symptoms?

A: By focusing on improving nutrition, exercise and overall health and on correcting any imbalances in the body. Some homeopathic doctors—including Andrew Lockie, M.D., and Nicola Geddes, M.D., authors of *The Women's Guide to Homeopathy*—prescribe HRT for menopausal women, particularly for those who have had a surgical menopause. At the same time, Lockie and Geddes are careful not to encourage women to use hormone therapy "as a substitute for adopting a healthy lifestyle," they write. The authors advise women to prepare for menopause by reevaluating their diet and exercise plans and by developing positive attitudes toward menopause.

Homeopathic physicians, or homeopaths, have more than 3,000 remedies in their lexicon, each designed to treat very specific complaints. And because each remedy or dose must be individualized to each woman, homeopaths don't like to recommend general therapies for menopausal women. Lockie and Geddes note that remedies exist that can be used as homeopathic HRT, but they believe these should be used only under the guidance of an experienced homeopath.

NATUROPATHY

Q: What can you tell me about naturopathy?

A: Naturopathy is a healing art that emphasizes the body's natural healing forces and makes use of massage, herbal therapy, homeopathy and a number of other alternative therapies to treat a range of conditions. Naturopathy uses a woman's medical history to make a diagnosis, supplemented by laboratory tests and other diagnostic techniques such as x-rays, scans and physicals. Once a diagnosis is made, the naturopath (a health professional who practices naturopathy) sets about restoring health by taking the whole woman into account, not just her symptoms. Naturopaths consider diet and nutrition essential to good health and advise women on the types of foods to eat, as well as those to avoid. Regular exercise is also considered essential to good health.

Q: How does a naturopath treat menopausal symptoms and menopause-related conditions?

A: Along with diet, nutrition and exercise, naturopathy uses herbs and botanical medicines, considered the cornerstone of naturopathic medicine (as well as of other alternative therapies). Let's take a look at osteoporosis as an example. To prevent or stop its progression, naturopaths devise a regimen of exercise, diet, vitamin and mineral supplementation, and botanical herbs. Michael Murray, N.D., and Joseph Pizzorno, N.D., writing in the *Encyclopedia of Natural Medicine,* propose a plan that consists of walking 45 to 60 minutes three to five times weekly; a diet high in fiber and low in fat and meat, with restricted intakes of refined carbohydrates, alcohol and carbonated beverages; and supplements of calcium, magnesium, vitamin B_{12}, folate and vitamin K, among others.

To treat atrophic vaginitis, Murray and Pizzorno recommend a low-fat, nutrient-rich diet with no refined foods or simple carbohydrates such as sugar; supplements of B-complex vitamins and vitamin E; topical vitamin E cream; and phytoestrogenic foods and herbs.

HERBAL MEDICINE

Q: What can you tell me about herbal medicine?

A: Herbal medicine is as old as humankind. It's a healing art that uses plants to treat and prevent illness. At one time, traditional and herbal medicine coexisted. Then mainstream medicine took over, after which herbal medicine was considered folk medicine or just plain quackery. But the fact is that all early medicines were vegetable in origin because the elaborate process of making synthetic compounds didn't exist. Today, herbal medicine is gaining in popularity and is recognized as an effective treatment for many conditions, including menopausal symptoms.

Q: Because herbal remedies seem to be available in many places, can I just go to the store and buy herbs to treat my symptoms?

A: Rather than diagnosing yourself, most alternative practitioners recommend that you get a specific, personalized botanical formula based on a diagnosis of your particular menopausal symptoms, medical history and overall health.

Herbalists claim that their remedies don't have the harmful side effects of modern medicines. While most herbs are safe in moderation, some can cause unexpected allergic or toxic reactions if taken in too large or too frequent doses. Be aware, too, that herbs can interact with medicines. It's wise to always consult your doctor or a respected herbalist for recommendations of formulas and dosages.

Q: Which herbs are most effective in easing menopausal discomforts?

A: Many herbs are thought to be effective in easing menopausal discomforts. They include dong quai, ginseng, black cohosh, false unicorn root, licorice root, anise, red clover, motherwort, chamomile, vitex and St. John's wort.

Herbs for Menopausal Symptoms

Q: What is dong quai?

A: Dong quai is a phytoestrogen, or plant estrogen, which, as you may recall from chapter 2, is a chemical that the body converts into estrogen. This herb has been prescribed by Chinese doctors for hundreds of years to help alleviate hot flashes, breast tenderness, sore joints, insomnia and anxiety. It's one of the most common herbs for treating "female complaints" in this country, as well as abroad.

Q: Is it effective?

A: Actually, there is debate as to how effective dong quai is. Studies have found that dong quai can help ease hot flashes and lower blood pressure by dilating blood vessels. Because of its ability to dilate blood vessels, the herb may have cardiovascular-protecting properties as well, notes Daniel B. Mowrey, Ph.D., in *Herbal Tonic Therapies.* Studies have also shown that the herb has pain-relieving properties.

In a small study of postmenopausal women, Bruce Ettinger, M.D., senior research investigator at Kaiser Permanente Medical Care Program in Oakland, California, analyzed dong quai for possible estrogenic effects. Ettinger concluded that the herb performed no differently than a placebo (an inactive substance). He cautioned, though, that in China, dong quai is traditionally mixed with several other herbs and not taken alone, as was the case in his study. In other words, dong quai may not be as effective in helping to relieve menopausal symptoms when used alone as it is when combined with other herbs. Ettinger is working with Chinese researchers to develop a new approach that would use more complicated herbal formulations, according to *Nutrition Science News.*

At present, no scientific evidence exists to confirm that dong quai relieves insomnia or anxiety.

Q: Are there side effects with dong quai?

A: Women with fibroids and women on blood-thinning drugs should not use dong quai. It may also make women more vulnerable to sunburn and dermatitis.

Q: I've heard of ginseng. What is it used for?

A: Another plant estrogen, ginseng is used by Chinese herbalists to treat menopausal discomforts, stimulate the immune system, normalize blood pressure and reduce cholesterol levels, writes Dee Ito in *Without Estrogen: Natural Remedies for Menopause and Beyond*. Ito notes that ginseng has an anticlotting effect that may reduce the risk of heart attack, has a protective effect on the liver and is rich in vitamins A, E and B_{12} and the mineral calcium.

Q: How effective is ginseng?

A: It depends on whom you talk to. Various Swedish studies, presented at the annual North American Menopause Society meeting in 1997, evaluated the effects of ginseng and got mixed results. One found that ginseng didn't differ from a placebo in its effects; another found that ginseng had no effect on vasomotor symptoms. But researchers from the Universities of Linkoping and Gothenburg in Sweden did report that ginseng can enhance well-being.

Q: Are there side effects with ginseng?

A: Possible side effects include allergy symptoms, asthma attacks, insomnia, breast soreness, increased blood pressure and disturbances in heart rhythm, cautions Michael Castleman in *The Healing Herbs*. Women with allergies, asthma, emphysema, fibrocystic breasts, high blood pressure, clotting problems or fever should not use ginseng.

Q: You mentioned black cohosh. What can you tell me about it?

A: Black cohosh is a phytoestrogenic herb, the root of which is used to relieve hot flashes, night sweats, vaginal dryness, incontinence, irritability, anxiety, headaches and depression.

Q: How effective is it?

A: Studies have shown that it alleviates most menopausal symptoms. In addition to easing hot flashes, the herb tones and strengthens pelvic muscles, improves digestion and relieves headaches, says Susun Weed in *Menopausal Years— The Wise Woman Way.*

Q: Are there side effects with black cohosh?

A: The Food and Drug Administration (FDA) states that black cohosh has no therapeutic value and warns that overdoses can cause dizziness, nausea, vomiting, headaches and a depressed heart rate, according to Castleman.

Q: What was the other herb that you mentioned— unicorn something?

A: You mean false unicorn root. The herb, a native North American plant, is also a phytoestrogen. Andrew Chevallier, in *The Encyclopedia of Medicinal Plants,* says that false unicorn "is a valuable remedy for menstrual problems and ovarian cysts and can also be very beneficial during menopause."

According to Ito, the root can lift depression, soothe headaches and stimulate the reproductive organs.

Q: Does false unicorn root have any side effects?

A: Unfortunately, there is little research on false unicorn root, including possible side effects. Don't exceed the recommended dosage prescribed by your health practitioner.

Q: I forgot the other herbs you mentioned. Can you refresh my memory?

A: Certainly—licorice root, anise, red clover, motherwort, chamomile, vitex and St. John's wort. Licorice root is a phytoestrogen that is used to treat hot flashes, vaginal dryness and sore joints. Ito says that it's often combined with sarsaparilla root because sarsaparilla contains progesterone and helps balance the effects of licorice. Increased energy levels and reduced stress are benefits that can be derived from licorice.

Q: How effective is licorice?

A: Researchers have found that licorice may help relieve vaginal dryness and hot flashes. To date, no conclusive study has been done. However, according to an article in *American Health,* the root's anti-inflammatory effects have been well proven.

Q: Are there side effects with licorice?

A: This herb may increase blood pressure and should be avoided by anyone with hypertension, kidney failure or cardiovascular disease. Large amounts of licorice root may cause swelling.

Q: You mentioned anise. How is it beneficial?

A: Because aniseed contains phytoestrogens, it may help relieve menopausal discomforts, says Castleman. He notes that the FDA considers anise to be safe, but high doses of the herb—several teaspoons—can cause nausea and vomiting.

Q: How is red clover helpful?

A: This herb can act like estrogen when taken in large quantities. According to Weed, red clover is a "calming reliever of menopausal distresses such as sore joints, anxiety and energy loss." The FDA considers red clover to be safe, though this plant can sometimes cause mild stomach upset or diarrhea.

Q: And what can you tell me about motherwort? How is it beneficial?

A: Motherwort is an herb that can aid in relieving palpitations (unusually fast heartbeats), which sometimes accompany hot flashes. It can also be used to help women wean themselves off HRT, says Diane Stein in *The Natural Remedy Book for Women*. In the book, Stein discusses how motherwort can ease the transition and keep the body from slipping into a state of hormonal imbalance.

Q: Does motherwort have any side effects?

A: According to Castleman, women with clotting disorders shouldn't use motherwort because of its potential anticlotting effects. Further, some women develop rashes from contact with this plant. Women who are taking sedatives and heart or blood pressure medications should avoid this herb. Other possible effects include diarrhea and stomach upset.

Q: I've heard a lot about chamomile. Isn't it used to calm?

A: You're right. Chamomile, often served as a tea, is a relaxant, according to *The Dictionary of Modern Herbalism.* As is true of lemon verbena, woodruff, hawthorn, hops and passionflower, chamomile may help menopausal women who are particularly anxious, agitated, restless and sleepless, say Lockie and Geddes.

Q: Does chamomile have side effects?

A: The FDA regards this herb as safe, but large amounts of highly concentrated preparations have caused nausea and vomiting. Other possible side effects include a rash from contact with the fresh plant. Rarely, chamomile may cause dangerous allergic reactions in people with allergies to ragweed.

Q: What does vitex do?

A: Vitex, also known as chasteberry, is thought to regulate the irregular periods of women who are perimenopausal. Studies have found that vitex changes the estrogen-progesterone ratio by increasing progesterone levels. This effect may help regulate a woman's period.

Vitex is a slow-acting herb. It may take up to three months of daily use to see results, says Weed.

Q: Are there any side effects with vitex?

A: Possible side effects include headaches, low sex drive and increased menstrual flow.

Q: I've heard of St. John's wort. How is it helpful?

A: St. John's wort may help relieve anxiety and mild to moderate depression, according to an article in the *Journal of the American Medical Association.* A few studies of short-term use have shown that St. John's wort is just as effective as low doses of certain antidepressants in treating depression. Whether St. John's wort is just as effective with long-term use is unknown, however.

Q: Are there side effects with St. John's wort?

A: No serious side effects have been reported, but some women may get upset stomachs. There may be increased sensitivity to the sun as well. St. John's wort may interact with amphetamines, diet pills, narcotics, tyrosine (an amino acid) supplements, nasal decongestants, antidepressants, asthma inhalers, and cold and allergy medications, warns Castleman.

Q: Are there any other herbs that may be helpful?

A: Yes. There are several herbs that can be used during and after menopause, including alfalfa for relieving water retention and bloating; garden sage for night sweats and hot flashes; juniper berries and buchu leaves for urinary incontinence; and wild Mexican yam (which contains natural progesterone) for anxiety.

Many alternative practitioners (including homeopathic, naturopathic and herbal) recommend herbs in combinations.

ACUPUNCTURE AND ACUPRESSURE

Q: I've seen acupuncture on television. Can you explain in more detail what it is?

A: Acupuncture is an ancient Chinese healing art in which very thin needles are inserted under the skin, at specific sites on the body, to treat illness and restore good health.

Chinese medicine teaches that in order to remain healthy, yin and yang (negative and positive forces) must be perfectly balanced and a life force known as chi must flow throughout the body. The chi flows along paths known as meridians (sets of invisible lines) and covers the body in set patterns. While meridians are not identical to the nervous system or circulatory system, they are thought to resemble those systems. When illness occurs, the acupuncturist (a practitioner of acupuncture) examines the meridians and carefully selects acupuncture sites. It is at these sites that needles are inserted.

Q: How does acupuncture help with menopausal symptoms?

A: Some women find that it helps relieve the severity and frequency of hot flashes and other vasomotor symptoms.

Q: You also mentioned acupressure, which sounds like acupuncture. Is it the same thing?

A: In some ways, it is. Acupressure is also a form of Chinese medicine. In this therapy, the fingers are used instead of needles to apply pressure along the meridians. By stimulating points along the meridians, acupressure encourages the life force to flow to various parts of the body.

Asian medical practitioners treat hot flashes by pressing "cooling points" on the feet and hands to balance body temperature, says Cathryn Bauer in *Acupressure for Everybody.*

BIOFEEDBACK

Q: What is biofeedback?

A: Biofeedback is a psychological therapy that uses the conscious mind to control involuntary body functions such as respiration, heartbeat and body temperature.

Q: How can this help with menopausal symptoms?

A: After being trained in biofeedback, some menopausal women are able to reduce the frequency and severity of their hot flashes. Biofeedback can also be used as a relaxation technique and has been used to treat stress headaches, migraines and back pain.

Q: Can anyone learn biofeedback?

A: Yes. But the techniques used to train someone have become very sophisticated. Often these techniques are learned at a medical center or at a clinic where certified instructors specialize in teaching biofeedback. Using high-tech equipment, the practitioner can monitor brain impulses and make them audible to the woman who is using biofeedback. By monitoring this electrical activity and listening to a series of beeps, the woman learns how to control the situation.

Q: Are there other alternative therapies for menopausal discomforts?

A: Yes. Other healing arts—including Chinese medicine, Ayurvedic medicine (a holistic healing art originating in India) and Bach flower remedies (a form of herbal medicine)—may have approaches to help you cope with menopausal discomforts.

CHOOSING AN ALTERNATIVE THERAPY AND PRACTITIONER

Q: I would like to try alternative therapy. But with so many choices, how do I know which one is right for me?

A: There are a few things you should consider. First, base your decision on what type of medical condition you have. For example, if you are experiencing hot flashes, naturopathy or herbal medicine may be a good choice. Second, choose something you're interested in. If the thought of acupuncture makes you tuck tail and run, it may not be right for you. Third, read as much as you can about the various therapies at your local library or health food store. Fourth, ask friends, family and coworkers about their experiences with a particular alternative therapy. Finally, ask your doctor for a recommendation. More and more health practitioners are becoming familiar with alternative therapies and support their patients' decisions to go that route.

Q: OK. How do I choose an alternative practitioner?

A: Once you've decided on the form of alternative therapy, you need to select a practitioner. First, find out if the field in which she practices requires a license in your state.

Q: But how do I find out that information?

A: Call your state department of professional and occupational licensure. You may have to contact the information operator at your state capital if this agency isn't listed in your telephone book. If the field of alternative medicine you've chosen does require a license, the licensure agency can give you the name of the licensing board that you can call for more details on the credentials of any potential practitioner.

The next step is to find a specific provider. Collect the names and addresses of practitioners in your area. Again, ask family, friends and other contacts for the names of practitioners they have used. Check your telephone directory for alternative practitioners—they're sometimes listed under the particular therapy. Another resource is the on-line service operated by the American Holistic Health Association, which provides practitioner referrals (see "Informational and Mutual-Aid Groups" at the end of this book).

Q: Is there anything specific I need to be aware of when it comes to finding an alternative practitioner?

A: For one thing, not all alternative therapy is standardized or regulated (but neither is much of mainstream medicine!). Keep the following issues in mind when narrowing your choices.

- *Unrealistic claims and promises.* Be leery of practitioners who make unrealistic claims and promises. Reputable alternative practitioners reject such outlandish assertions.

- *Licensure and certification.* Does the practitioner have a license and certificate as required in her particular field of alternative medicine? Licensing and certification are never absolute assurances of quality, but they prove to you that the person has completed an approved training program that has met certain qualifications.

- *Accreditation.* Look for any evidence that the practitioner has been recognized by her peer group or has received awards. Professional organizations may accredit members who have completed additional training or passed special examinations.

- *Excessive return visits.* Watch out for a treatment regimen that has you returning three to four times a week for many weeks. Reputable practitioners will schedule you for return visits only when such visits are truly necessary.

- *Limited hospital privileges.* Check with your local hospital to find out if the alternative practitioner you're interested in has admitting privileges and if there are any conditions or limitations on those privileges.

- *Free services and contracts.* Be leery of free services, which are often gimmicks to lure you into an office. Once you're there, you may find your wallet a little lighter because of additional treatments.

- *Referral patterns.* Ask about referrals to other professionals, including M.D.'s and D.O.'s, if your medical problem is beyond the practitioner's skills. An alternative practitioner who makes light of the need for a referral may be someone who doesn't know her limitations.

- *History of complaints.* Again, check with your state department of professional and occupational licensure to find out if complaints have been filed against a practitioner. Contact your local Better Business Bureau and local courts for any complaints or malpractice cases brought against the practitioner and determine what happened in any cases on record.

Q: Can I go to a medical doctor for alternative therapy?

A: Yes. Some alternative practitioners are also M.D.'s or D.O.'s, meaning that they combine traditional scientific (allopathic) medicine with alternative therapies. A woman who wants to explore an alternative treatment for menopause-related conditions but who doesn't want to abandon the mainstream medical system may wish to consult one of these doctors.

Q: I see now that there are many treatment choices for menopausal symptoms and many prevention methods for menopause-related conditions. Is there anything you'd like to add?

A: We wish we could say that everything a woman needs to know about nonhormonal therapy and HRT lies within the pages of this book, but that would be a false promise. More research is needed to further prove or disprove the current facts about the forms of therapy we've covered, especially HRT.

MENOPAUSE: LOOKING AT THE GREATER WHOLE

Q: Menopause seems like the final phase of life, and that saddens and frightens me. Do other women feel the same?

A: You're not alone. Many American women feel that menopause marks the end of life—no doubt due to American culture, which typically depicts older women as weak, nonsexual, unhappy and unattractive. But as more

American women than ever before in our country's history enter menopause, they're changing negative attitudes toward menopause.

Q: How so?

A:
By refusing to accept inhibiting cultural attitudes toward menopause, women encourage all people (including their partners) to reexamine the stereotype that implies postmenopausal women have nothing to offer society.

Q: But how can women change attitudes?

A:
That process begins with the individual woman. More women are recognizing what has been a part of the belief system of many indigenous societies—that menopause is not just a physiological change. Many cultures, past and present, see menopause as a rite of passage—a spiritual, emotional and psychological transition—and as a time when a woman enters a powerful stage of life. Judith K. Brown, coeditor of *In Her Prime: New Views of Middle-Aged Women,* notes that women of many indigenous societies move into positions of power and prestige after menopause.

And as more women recognize the impact of other positive cultural attitudes toward menopause, they can incorporate these beliefs into their own philosophies and create their own rites of passage that honor menopause.

INFORMATIONAL AND MUTUAL-AID GROUPS

Acupressure Institute
1533 Shattuck Ave.
Berkeley, CA 94709
510-845-1059

Provides free catalog of books, videotapes and acupressure tools.

American Association of Naturopathic Physicians
601 Valley St., #105
Seattle, WA 98109
206-298-0126

Provides national referral directory of all U.S. members and informational brochure on naturopathic medicine for $5 prepaid.

American Botanical Council
P.O. Box 144345
Austin, TX 78714
512-331-8868

Publishes HerbalGram *magazine and booklets on herbs. Offers reprints of scientific articles. Sells hard-to-locate books on herbalism.*

American Cancer Society
1599 Clifton Rd., N.E.
Atlanta, GA 30329
404-320-3333
800-ACS-2345

Publishes free materials on cancer prevention and treatment.

American College of Nurse-Midwives
818 Connecticut Ave., N.W., Suite 900
Washington, DC 20006
202-728-9860

Provides listings of nurse-midwives by state and pamphlets and brochures.

American College of Obstetricians and Gynecologists
409 12th St., S.W.
Washington, DC 20024
202-638-5577

Publishes free informational pamphlets. Provides lists of board-certified physicians.

American Heart Association
7272 Greenville Ave.
Dallas, TX 75231
214-373-6300

Publishes materials on heart disease prevention and treatment.

American Holistic Health Association
P.O. Box 17400
Anaheim, CA 92817-7400
714-779-6152
www.healthy.net/ahha/

Publishes newsletter and other informational materials on complementary medicine. Provides referrals to holistic practitioners.

Biofeedback Certification Institute of America
10200 W. 44th Ave., Suite 310
Wheat Ridge, CO 80033
303-420-2902

Runs the major certification program for biofeedback practitioners. Provides referrals to certified local practitioners.

Boston Women's Health Book Collective
Box 192
West Somerville, MA 02144
617-625-0271
617-625-0277

Maintains consumer health library open to the public by appointment. Publishes books and brochures on women's health issues. Send a business-size, self-addressed, stamped envelope for a list of publications, services and current activities.

Cancer Information Service
of the National Cancer Institute
NCI/NIH, Bldg. 31, 10A16
9000 Rockville Pike
Bethesda, MD 20892-2580
800-4-CANCER

Provides free cancer information service. Staffed by trained counselors. Offers detailed information on 150 types of cancer. Also offers referrals to hospitals, support groups and information on financial aid.

Center for Medical Consumers
237 Thompson St.
New York, NY 10012
212-674-7105

Provides medical library and publishes HealthFacts, *a newsletter that presents controversial health care issues.*

A Friend Indeed
Box 1710
Champlain, NY 12919-1710
514-843-5730

Monthly newsletter with information on latest research on menopause and other health topics for women.

Menopause News
800-241-MENO

Newsletter with information on latest research and developments in treating menopausal symptoms.

National Center for Homeopathy
801 N. Fairfax St., Suite 306
Alexandria, VA 22314
703-548-7790

Provides packet to consumers for $7, which includes general information and annual directory of homeopathic practitioners and study groups.

National Certification Commission for Acupuncture and Oriental Medicine
11 Canal Center Plaza, Suite 200
Alexandria, VA 22314
703-548-9004

Provides state lists of certified acupuncturists for $3 prepaid. Send your request in writing.

National Osteoporosis Foundation
1150 17th St., N.E., Suite 500
Washington, DC 20036
202-223-2226
800-223-9994

Publishes pamphlets and offers copies of research articles on the subject of osteoporosis.

National Women's Health Network
514 10th St., N.W., Suite 400
Washington, DC 20004
202-347-1140

Offers packets of resource materials on general or specific topics (available for $8). Write for a free directory of topics and a one-page brief on your particular health concern.

North American Menopause Society
P.O. Box 94527
Cleveland, OH 44101-4527
216-844-8748

Provides information on menopause. Offers lists of menopause treatment centers and free quarterly newsletter.

GLOSSARY

Absolute contraindication: Situation or medical condition that prohibits the use of hormone replacement therapy.

Acupressure: Healing art in which the fingers are used to apply pressure to specific sites on the body to treat illness and restore health.

Acupuncture: Healing art in which thin needles are inserted under the skin at specific sites on the body to treat illness and restore health.

Adrenal gland: One of two glands situated near the kidneys that produce many hormones, including epinephrine (adrenaline), androstenedione (later converted into estrone), testosterone, mineralocorticoids and glucocorticoids.

Amenorrhea: Lack of menstruation; abnormal cessation of the menstrual cycle.

Androgen: Substance (such as a hormone) that produces masculine characteristics in the body.

Angiotensin: Chemical that causes blood vessels to narrow.

Antihypertensive: Drug used to lower blood pressure.

Artificial menopause: See **surgical menopause**.

Atherosclerosis: Condition in which the inner layers of artery walls become thick and irregular due to deposits of fat, cholesterol and other substances.

Atrophic: Degenerative.

Atrophic vaginitis: Shrinking, drying and lessening elasticity of vaginal tissues after menopause; can cause discomfort during sex and lead to more frequent vaginal infections.

Bartholin's gland: One of two small glands inside the vaginal opening that secrete drops of fluid during sexual arousal.

Biofeedback: Psychological therapy that uses the conscious mind to control involuntary body functions such as respiration, heartbeat and body temperature.

Bioflavonoid: See **flavonoid**.

Bisphosphonate: Drug that can prevent bone loss.

Bone mass: Total amount of bone tissue.

Bone resorption: Process by which bones dissolve and lose calcium.

Breakthrough bleeding: Unplanned, abnormal uterine bleeding between menstrual periods.

Breast cancer: Cancerous tumor of the breast tissue.

Buccal estrogen: Estrogen administered by means of a tablet placed against the cheek so that the estrogen is absorbed through the mucous membranes into the bloodstream; not currently approved for use in the United States.

Calcitonin: Hormone that decreases calcium in the bloodstream and that is thought to help bones absorb calcium.

Calcitriol: Active form of vitamin D in the body; drug that appears to be an effective osteoporosis medication and that is thought to help bones absorb calcium and phosphorus.

Cerebrovascular accident: Stroke.

Cervix: Bottom of the uterus that extends into the vagina.

Climacteric: See **menopause**.

Clitoris: Part of the female external sex organs that is highly sensitive to touch.

Collagen: Protein that provides structural support for skin, bone, cartilage and connective tissue.

Combination therapy: Form of hormone replacement therapy in which a woman takes progestin in addition to one of the forms of estrogen; also known as combined hormone therapy.

Combined hormone therapy (CHT): See **combination therapy**.

Conjugated equine estrogen: Estrogen in pill form derived from the urine of pregnant mares.

Continuous combined therapy: Form of hormone replacement therapy in which a woman takes a small amount of progestin along with estrogen every day of the month.

Continuous sequential therapy: Form of hormone replacement therapy in which a woman takes estrogen continuously, every day of the month, with progestin taken for 12 to 14 days of the month (from day 12 through day 25).

Contraindication: Symptom or condition that makes a particular procedure or treatment inadvisable.

Corpus luteum: Ruptured follicle's scar tissue that temporarily manufactures progesterone.

Cortical bone: Dense and hard tissue; outer layer of bone.

CT (computerized tomography) scan: Radiography that uses a computer to create a 3-D picture of a body structure.

Cyclic combined therapy: Form of hormone replacement therapy in which a woman takes estrogen and low-dosage progestin for 25 days each month.

Cyclic sequential therapy: Form of hormone replacement therapy in which a woman takes estrogen for 21 or 25 days of the month, adding progestin to the estrogen for the last 10 or 14 days.

Dilatation and curettage (D&C): Surgical procedure in which the cervix is dilated (widened) so that the physician can scrape and remove the endometrium with a curette (a spoon-shaped instrument).

Dual-energy x-ray absorptiometry (DEXA): Test that measures the density of bone tissue in the wrist, arm, spine, hip or thighbone.

Dual-photon absorptiometry (DPA): Test that measures the density of bone tissue in the spine, hip or thighbone.

Embolism: Blockage of a blood vessel caused by an embolus.

Embolus: Blood clot, object, bit of tissue or gas in a blood vessel.

Endocrine system: Network of glands that manufacture hormones and release them into the bloodstream.

Endometrial biopsy: Microscopic examination of a sample of tissue from the lining of the uterus.

Endometrial cancer: Cancerous tumor of the uterine lining.

Endometriosis: Condition in which cells from the endo-metrium (uterine lining) migrate outside the uterus and grow on other organs in the abdomen.

Endometrium: Lining of the uterus.

ERT: See **estrogen replacement therapy**.

Esterified estrogen: Form of natural estrogen used in hormone replacement therapy.

Estradiol: Most potent form of estrogen; produced by the ovaries.

Estriol: Weak estrogen produced in the female body.

Estrogen: One of several hormones that control the reproductive process in the female body. The three types of estrogen are estradiol, estrone and estriol.

Estrogen replacement therapy (ERT): Medical treatment to replace some of the estrogen lost after menopause; form of hormone replacement therapy.

Estrogen therapy (ET): See **estrogen replacement therapy (ERT)**.

Estrone: Low-level estrogen produced in the body's fatty tissues.

Estropipate: Synthetic estrogen used in hormone replacement therapy.

Fallopian tube: One of two thin tubes that capture eggs as they leave the ovaries and transport them to the uterus.

Fibroid: Noncancerous growth in uterine muscle tissue.

Flavonoid: Colorful and aromatic compound found in fruit and which is a weak plant estrogen; also known as a bioflavonoid. See **phytoestrogen**.

Follicle: Sac or tubular gland in the ovary containing an immature egg.

Follicle-stimulating hormone (FSH): Hormone released by the pituitary gland to stimulate the ovaries to produce estrogen and to encourage the egg follicles in the ovaries to mature.

Follicle-stimulating hormone (FSH) test: Blood test that measures the amount of follicle-stimulating hormone; used to help make a diagnosis of menopause.

Formication: Sensation of something crawling on the skin; one vasomotor symptom of menopause.

FSH: See **follicle-stimulating hormone**.

FSH test: See **follicle-stimulating hormone test**.

Genitourinary symptom: Symptom occurring months or years after menopause in response to low estrogen levels; includes more frequent urination, vaginal dryness, vaginal infections and urinary tract infections.

Gonadotropin: Hormone that causes the ovaries and testes to act.

Gonadotropin-releasing hormone: Hormone released by the hypothalamus that tells the pituitary gland to release one of two gonadotropins—follicle-stimulating hormone and luteinizing hormone.

HDL: See **high-density lipoprotein**.

Heart disease: Abnormal condition of the heart or of the heart and circulation.

Herbal medicine: Healing art that uses plants to prevent and cure illness.

High-density lipoprotein (HDL): So-called good cholesterol that helps escort cholesterol and other lipids from the body. High levels are linked to reduced risk of heart disease.

Homeopathic medicine: See **homeopathy**.

Homeopathy: System of medicine that treats illness by using natural medicines that stimulate a person's own healing powers while avoiding harmful side effects; also known as homeopathic medicine.

Hormone: Naturally occurring chemical in one part of the body that produces physical effects in another part of the body.

Hormone replacement therapy (HRT): Medical treatment to replace some of the estrogen and progesterone lost after menopause.

Hot flash: Menopausal symptom characterized by a sensation of intense warmth and a pink flush in the head, neck and upper body that can last from a few seconds to an hour; also known as a hot flush.

Hot flush: See **hot flash**.

HRT: See **hormone replacement therapy**.

Hyperplasia: Proliferation of cells in the uterine lining that can lead to uterine cancer.

Hypertension: High blood pressure.

Hypothalamus: Small but powerful gland in the brain that oversees the reproductive endocrine system, as well as other body functions.

Hysterectomy: Surgical removal of the uterus.

Implanted subcutaneous estrogen pellet: Estrogen administered by means of pellets or capsules surgically implanted under the skin; not currently approved for use in the United States.

Isoflavone: Colorless chemical compound occurring as a form of plant estrogen. See **phytoestrogen**.

Kegel exercise: Exercise that strengthens muscles that control urination; also called pubococcygeus exercise, after the muscles affected.

Labia majora: Outer lips of the vulva.

Labia minora: Inner lips of the vulva.

LDL: See **low-density lipoprotein**.

LH: See **luteinizing hormone**.

Lignan: One of several plant estrogens. See **phytoestrogen**.

Lipid: Greasy substance such as fatty acid or wax; stored in the body for use as energy reserves.

Low-density lipoprotein (LDL): So-called bad cholesterol. High levels have been linked to increased risk of heart disease.

Luteinizing hormone (LH): Gonadotropin hormone that causes ovulation.

Mastalgia: Breast tenderness or pain.

Mediator: Substance made of fatty acids that helps hormones carry out their jobs.

Menarche: First menstrual period; signifies the beginning of menstruation and the start of the reproductive years.

Menopause: Normal and complete cessation of menstrual cycles; in everyday usage, the months before and years after the last period.

Menstrual cycle: Repeating cycle of change in the endometrium (lining of the uterus), preparing it for the implantation and support of a fertilized egg; ends in menstruation if no egg is fertilized.

Menstruation: Sloughing off of the built-up uterine lining that occurs if conception does not take place.

Micronized estradiol: Form of estrogen sold in pills.

Naturopathy: Healing art that emphasizes using the body's natural healing forces.

Night sweat: Menopausal symptom characterized by excessive, drenching sweat that occurs during the night.

Nocturia: Excessive urination at night.

Oophorectomy: Surgical removal of the ovaries.

Opiate: Chemical that induces rest and quiets uneasiness.

Oral contraceptive: Birth control pill.

Osteopenia: Low bone mass.

Osteoporosis: Condition in which bones gradually lose their mineral content, becoming porous, thin and fragile.

Ovarian cancer: Cancerous tumor of the ovary.

Ovary: One of two female endocrine glands that contain unfertilized egg cells; produces the hormones estrogen, progesterone and testosterone.

Ovulation: Release of an egg from the ovary.

Ovum: Female reproductive cell.

Palpitation: Pounding or rapid racing of the heart.

Perimenopause: Years immediately before menopause.

Photo absorptiometry scan: Radioactive scan that evaluates bone density to check for osteoporosis.

Phytoestrogen: Chemical that the body converts into estrogen; also known as plant estrogen. Foods high in phytoestrogens include soy products (soybeans, tofu and miso), papaya and yams. Lesser amounts can be found in apples, brown rice, carrots, green beans, peas, potatoes, red beans, sesame seeds, whole wheat and rye.

Pituitary gland: Pebble-size endocrine gland that works in conjunction with the hypothalamus to regulate hormone production in the body.

Plant estrogen: See **phytoestrogen**.

Postmenopause: After menopause.

Premature menopause: Menopause before age 40, regardless of the reason.

Progesterone: Female sex hormone produced by the ovaries during the second half of the menstrual cycle.

Progesterone challenge test: Test to determine whether irregular menstrual periods or hyperplasia is caused by insufficient progesterone levels.

Progestin: Synthetic or natural form of progesterone.

Prostaglandin: Chemical mediator that causes contractions in the uterus.

Puberty: Period during which sexual maturity is attained.

Pubococcygeus exercise: See **Kegel exercise**.

QCT: See **quantitative computerized tomography**.

Quantitative computerized tomography (QCT scan or CT scan): Test to measure trabecular bone within the vertebrae and create a 3-D image of the spine.

Radiographic absorptiometry (RA): X-ray taken of the hand to measure density of bone tissue, detect fractures and help the health care practitioner diagnose osteoporosis.

Raloxifene: Drug that acts like estrogen on bone tissue. See **selective estrogen receptor modulator (SERM).**

Relative contraindication: Situation or medical condition under which hormone replacement therapy should be used with great care and medical supervision.

Risedronate: Drug to prevent further bone loss in women with osteoporosis.

Salmon calcitonin: Drug to prevent further bone loss in women with osteoporosis.

Sedative: Drug that decreases activity, relieves anxiety and produces calm.

Selective estrogen receptor modulator (SERM): Drug that acts like estrogen on bone tissue but does not affect the reproductive organs.

Single-photon absorptiometry (SPA): Outmoded test designed to measure density of bone tissue in the wrist or heel.

Sodium fluoride: Drug used to treat osteoporosis.

Surgical menopause: Menopause caused by surgical removal of the ovaries; also known as artificial menopause.

Testosterone: Androgen (male hormone) produced in small amounts by the ovaries.

Thromboembolic disease: Condition that causes blood-clotting problems.

Thrombophlebitis: Blood clot and inflammation in a deep vein, such as in a leg.

Thrombus: Blood clot.

Trabecular bone: Porous bone tissue.

Tranquilizer: Drug that calms, lessens anxiety and tension and induces drowsiness.

Transdermal estrogen: Estrogen administered by means of an adhesive patch applied to the skin.

Unopposed estrogen: Estrogen given alone without any other hormone.

Urethra: Tube that drains urine from the bladder.

Urinary incontinence: Involuntary leaking of urine.

Uterus: Female organ composed of muscle and glandular tissue; the womb.

Vagina: Resilient, muscular tract that extends from the uterus to the vulva.

Vaginal estrogen cream: Estrogen administered by means of an applicator that dispenses a measured amount of cream into the vagina.

Vaginal ring implant: Estrogen delivered by means of a ring inserted in the vagina and left there to slowly release set amounts of estrogen every 24 hours.

Vaginal suppository: Oval-shaped cone of medication inserted into the vagina, where it releases medicine to be absorbed into the body.

Vasomotor symptom: Menopausal symptom that relates to the nerves and muscles that open and close blood vessels; includes hot flashes and night sweats.

Vulva: External genitals of the female that include labia majora, labia minora, clitoris, and urinary and vaginal openings.

Withdrawal bleeding: Periodic uterine bleeding that occurs in some women taking certain combination forms of hormone replacement therapy; similar to a menstrual period.

SUGGESTED READING

Books and Booklets

American College of Obstetricians and Gynecologists. *Hormone Replacement Therapy.* Educational Bulletin Number 247 (May 1998).

Bauer, Cathryn. *Acupressure for Everybody: Gentle, Effective Relief for More Than 100 Common Ailments.* New York: Holt, 1991.

Bonnick, Sydney Lou, M.D., F.A.C.P. *The Osteoporosis Handbook,* 2nd ed. Dallas: Taylor Publishing, 1997.

Carr, Bruce R., M.D., and Jean D. Wilson, M.D. "Disorders of the Ovary and Female Reproductive Tract." In *Harrison's Principles of Internal Medicine,* 12th ed. Edited by Kurt J. Isselbacher, M.D., et al. New York: McGraw-Hill, 1994.

Castleman, Michael. *The Healing Herbs: The Ultimate Guide to the Curative Powers of Nature's Medicines.* New York: Bantam Books, 1995.

Cherry, Sheldon H., M.D., and Carolyn D. Runowicz, M.D. *The Menopause Book: A Guide to Health and Well-Being for Women After Forty.* New York: Macmillan, 1995.

Chevallier, Andrew. *The Encyclopedia of Medicinal Plants.* New York: DK Publishing, 1996.

Greenwood, Sadja, M.D. *Menopause, Naturally: Preparing for the Second Half of Life.* Volcano, Calif.: Volcano Press, 1996.

Heaney, Robert P., M.D., and M. Janet Barger-Lux. *Calcium and Common Sense.* New York: Doubleday, 1990.

Ito, Dee. *Without Estrogen: Natural Remedies for Menopause and Beyond.* New York: Carol Southern Books, 1995.

Lockie, Andrew, M.D., and Nicola Geddes, M.D. *The Women's Guide to Homeopathy.* New York: St. Martin's Press, 1994.

Love, Susan M., M.D., with Karen Lindsey. *Dr. Susan Love's Hormone Book.* New York: Random House, 1998.

McIlwain, Harris, M.D., and Debra Fulghum Bruce. *The Osteoporosis Cure.* New York: Avon Books, 1998.

Mishell, Daniel R., Jr., M.D. "Menopause." In *Conn's Current Therapy, 1995.* Edited by Robert E. Rakel, M.D. Philadelphia: W.B. Saunders, 1995.

Mowrey, Daniel B., Ph.D. *Herbal Tonic Therapies.* New Canaan, Conn.: Keats Publishing, 1993.

Murray, Michael, N.D, and Joseph Pizzorno, N.D. *Encyclopedia of Natural Medicine,* 2nd ed. Rocklin, Calif.: Prima Publishing, 1997.

Utian, Wulf H., M.D., Ph.D., and Ruth S. Jacobowitz. *Managing Your Menopause.* New York: Simon & Schuster, 1990.

Weed, Susun S. *Menopausal Years—The Wise Woman Way.* Woodstock, N.Y.: Ash Tree Publishing, 1992.

Articles

American Dietetic Association. "Translating the Science Behind the Dietary Reference Intakes." *Journal of the American Dietetic Association* 98, no. 7 (July 1998): 756.

Atkinson, Holly, M.D. "Preventing Osteoporosis." *Health News* 4, no. 3 (March 10, 1998): 1-2.

Barrett-Connor, Elizabeth, M.D. "Risks and Benefits of Replacement Estrogen." *Annual Review of Medicine* 43 (1992): 239-51.

Beral, V., et al. "Breast Cancer and Hormone Replacement Therapy." *Lancet* 350, no. 9084 (October 11, 1997): 1047-60.

Bowman, Marjorie A. "New Developments in Family Medicine." *Journal of the American Medical Association* 279, no. 18 (May 13, 1998): 1437-38.

Carroll, Linda. "Researchers Test Efficacy of Commonly Used Herbal Remedies for Menopause." *Nutrition Science News* 3, no. 3 (March 1998): 107.

Consumers Union. "Estrogen Therapy: Clearer Risks, Broader Benefits." *Consumer Reports on Health* 10, no. 5 (May 1998): 1-5.

Grodstein, Francine, Sc.D., et al. "Postmenopausal Hormone Therapy and Mortality." *New England Journal of Medicine* 336, no. 25 (June 19, 1997): 1769-75.

Grodstein, Francine, Sc.D., et al. "Postmenopausal Hormone Use and Risk for Colorectal Cancer and Adenoma." *Annals of Internal Medicine* 128, no. 9 (May 1, 1998): 705-13.

Karf, David B. "Prevention of Nonvertebral Fractures by Alendronate: A Meta-Analysis." *Journal of the American Medical Association* 277, no. 14 (April 9, 1997): 1159-65.

Kushing, Karla L., M.S. "Risks of Endometrial Cancer in Relation to Use of Low-Dose, Unopposed Estrogens." *Obstetrics and Gynecology* 91, no. 1 (January 1998): 35-39.

Province, Michael A., Ph.D., et al. "A Preplanned Meta-Analysis of the FICSIT Trials." *Journal of the American Medical Association* 273, no. 17 (May 3, 1995): 1341-48.

Shaw, Elizabeth. "What's Proven, What's Not: Natural Menopause Remedies." *American Health* 16, no. 8 (October 1997): 51.

Yaffe, Kristine, M.D., et al. "Estrogen Therapy in Postmenopausal Women: Effects on Cognitive Function and Dementia." *Journal of the American Medical Association* 279, no. 9 (March 4, 1998): 688-95.

Zacks, Rebecca. "Hormone Replacement Therapy." *Scientific American Presents: Women's Health* 9, no. 2 (Summer 1998): 82-85.

INDEX